Heidelberg
Science
Library

D0863619

W. W. Spradlin
P. B. Porterfield

Human Biosociology

From Cell to Culture

Springer-Verlag
New York
Heidelberg
Berlin

Wilford Wayne Spradlin, M.D.
Patricia Bavely Porterfield, M.S.W.
Department of Behavioral Medicine and Psychiatry
University of Virginia School of Medicine
Charlottesville, Virginia 22901

Library of Congress Cataloging in Publication Data

Spradlin, Wilford W
    Human biosociology.

    (Heidelberg science library)
    Includes index.
    1. Personality.   2.   Interpersonal relations.
3.   Social psychology.   4.   Social systems.
5.   Psychobiology.   I.   Porterfield, P. B., joint
author.   II.   Title.   III.   Series.
BF698.S66   155   78-31871

© 1979 by Springer-Verlag New York Inc.

Printed in the United States of America

9 8 7 6 5 4 3 2 1

ISBN 0-387-90350-X Springer-Verlag New York Heidelberg Berlin

ISBN 3-540-90350-X Springer-Verlag Berlin Heidelberg New York

To Katie and Charles Spradlin,
Lisa, David, Diane, and Cara Porterfield

Preface

There is growing evidence that an amalgamation of systems theories and communication and information theories will become the leading conceptual model for addressing human behavior. In this book we have used a theoretical frame which focuses on the coding, storage, and movement of information within and among open systems. We believe this to be a productive working concept which allows the student of human behavior to avoid the mind/body dichotomy. This conceptual framework also allows the integration of the biologic and sociologic aspects of human behavior. Using this theoretical model we may see science and art as a continuum of imaginative ways of organizing information.

Hence, the primary aim of this text is to provide a conceptual frame for students of human behavior which utilizes systems theories and information and communication theories in an integrated approach which is both theoretical and practical. It is written for the student in the behavioral sciences who may be planning a career in medicine, social work, psychology, nursing, guidance and counseling, the ministry, or other health and service professions. In addition, students in biology, sociology, and philosophy may benefit from this conceptual approach. It is also written for the practitioner who is currently delivering counseling and other health services to a variety of clientele.

Unfortunately, systems theories and information theories are often presented in a highly technical fashion using mathematical formulas which discourage many students and make the theories appear rather impersonal, mechanical, and detached. This book is not weighted with mathematical formulations and complex diagrams. Terminology has been simplified. Words such as equifinality and isomorphism that might alienate those with limited backgrounds in systems theories are omitted. Descriptions of mass and energy carriers of information which are emphasized in more comprehensive texts have been largely omitted in order to avoid unnecessary complexity.

We have attempted to make the study of information flow among individuals more personal by the use of vignettes. The vignettes usually supply only one side of a conversation or confrontation. This encourages the reader to supply his own retorts drawn from his life's experiences and from his understanding of similar situations. With this format which requires reader or subjective participation, we have attempted to avoid the distorting illusion of objective, detached observer which is evoked in many texts by formal case histories. The use of these vignettes further emphasizes the ways in which information interdigitates within and among open systems.

The questions given at the ends of Chapters 1 through 11 are designed to guide the reader in remembering the more crucial points in the material. Each question can be answered directly from the text and is not written to be misleading or difficult.

It is the hope of the authors that this brief presentation will inspire the reader to continue his study of the concepts introduced therein and that he will attempt to utilize some of them in his professional career.

Acknowledgments

We would like to acknowledge the following persons who helped us in the development of this project:

Dr. William Hobbs, Assistant Professor of Psychiatry, University of Virginia, Dr. David J. Withersty, Associate Professor of Psychiatry, West Virginia University School of Medicine, Morgantown, West Virginia, and Mr. Don Badger, social worker, Wake County Medical Center, Raleigh, North Carolina, who unselfishly spent many hours with us in critiquing our conceptual frames.

Mr. Phillip Paulucci, Instructor of Sociology, Mercyhurst College, Erie, Pennsylvania, who utilized portions of our manuscript in his behavioral science courses to test their effectiveness.

The Springer-Verlag staff, for their kind and enthusiastic encouragement.

Ms. Judy White, who has worked diligently and good-naturedly in the preparation and typing of this manuscript.

Contents

12

Evolution of a Systems Theory of Self and Society   181

Introduction

The way each individual comprehends the world is dependent on the conceptual framework that individual uses to organize incoming information. These conceptual frames of reference are biased by various learning experiences. Each discipline biases its students differently. Sociologists may comprehend the human condition differently from biologists because they are guided by their teachers and their colleagues to act or react in a certain manner to a given set of data, a manner utilized because it more nearly satisfies the sociologist's self-concept. These differences in concept formation will bias subsequent observations.

To understand ourselves as human entities and within our families and larger social structures, we may study anything along the continuum from cell to the cultures within which we live. The biologist might begin with the cell, whereas the sociologist might begin with the individual, the family, and the culture. Human behavior is the field that serves as a common denominator for the sociologist and the biologist. Through a biosocial approach, genetic, physiologic, psychologic, interpersonal, and social phenomena can be fitted into the same conceptual framework.

Human Biosociology is designed for the student in the biologic and sociologic sciences who is interested in the world, the human animal, and the human social condition "from cell to culture." It is not written to solve clinical or social problems, but rather to permit a different perception of ourselves and our place in the universe—to raise more questions than it answers.

This volume is a theoretical approach to the study of humanity that is general and flexible enough to incorporate many aspects of human behavior. It is a systems approach drawn from many existing theories, especially from general systems theory, information theory, communications theories, and learning theory.

One of the most pernicious problems confronting education is the premature imposition of a problem-solving set on any new system of ideas. Students and faculty often distort the learning process by the overt or covert thesis of, "Learn this so you will be able to. . . ." Learning becomes a "how to" exercise and any theoretical frame is first scrutinized as to what practical value it has. Students want to know if what is being taught will solve problems. If it will not, it is of no use. In relation to a particular book—if it is not pragmatic in its approach, why read it?

Students want to prepare for the work world, to get a job as soon as they graduate, to be able to "make it" economically as fast as possible. Most are no longer eager to learn just for the sake of learning, to consider an idea just because it is there, to see but not to try to solve.

Practicality is certainly a valid rationale for human endeavor, and all learning is in some sense a problem-solving activity. However, if learning is constricted to solving practical problems of our present situations, we may sacrifice a broader base of understanding that would be of value in solving problems that are at present unforeseen.

Many college students would smile, perhaps condescendingly at a question from an illiterate, mildly retarded tenant farmer who asked, "What do you want all that book learning for?" followed by the self-justifying statement, "I never went to school in my life and I get along all right."

Why should we smile? The statement is correct. The tenant farmer survives, works, eats, sleeps, has sex, enjoys watching television, etc. The student might state that these "essentials" are not enough—he or she wants a richer life. Yet, many students pose the tenant farmer's question to each course they select—"What good is it? Will it help me get a job, make a better salary, find easier work, get more rest, more sex, more passive entertainment?"

Learning for the pleasure of learning or attempting to understand without first asking, "Why understand?" has become somewhat rare in our technologically oriented educational systems. This is especially true in those educational programs focused on studying the human animal. Students want reassurance that educational programs will solve human problems as they perceive them prior to the learning situation. Yet, an open approach to understanding man in his environment might provide a new perspective of man's condition and perhaps better problem-solving capabilities than educational programs biased at onset to solve practical problems.

There is no guarantee. Perhaps the gamble is too great. But then again, perhaps the rewards are even greater. As educators, may we once again be persuaded that teaching students to ask questions is the greater goal.

The world runs for all to read. We go about and many of us are glad at times. Natural knowledge we commonly account a joyous thing; but it is clearly a saddening thing as well. Nature is like a music to which two friends can listen and both be moved and yet each by a different train of thought.

And the pursuit whose quest is Nature's understanding, has this among its rewards, that as it progresses its truth is testable. Truth is a 'value.' The quest itself therefore is in a measure its own satisfaction. We receive the lesson that our advance knowledge is of asymptotic type, even as continually approaching so continually without arrival. The satisfaction shall therefore be eternal.

—Sir Charles Sherrington, 1940
Man on His Nature

1 Basic Concepts

When it comes to atoms, language can be used only as in poetry. The poet, too, is not nearly so concerned with describing facts as with creating images.

Niels Bohr (2)

Man's Concept of the Universe

Throughout the universe there seems to be a constant changing, a simultaneous merging and parting, waxing and waning, coming together and separating of substrates to create unique entities which then dissolve into a more general solution. We say "seems to be" because that is only one way to perceive the universe, a way we can accept because it fits our present way of thinking. We cannot say, "Throughout the universe there *is* . . ." because that would suggest a certainty we cannot assume. We must continually remind ourselves that every conceptual model or term we utilize to help us describe phenomena depends on our present point of view and, therefore, contains distortions.

We must warn ourselves against the hazards of concrete or materialistic thinking. Scientific study can focus only on man's observations as its true object and not on any so-called realities of nature (6). All of our concepts must, then, be viewed as relative rather than absolute.

So we begin by *assuming* that there is an ebb and flow in the universe. In our search for a common denominator in this ebb and flow of being we conceptualize certain phenomena that we call mass and energy in a lattice of space and time. Perhaps there are more basic phenomena for which we at present have no concepts.

All these different parts are the constituents of the universe. They combine different ways at different times to make up series of relationships that we call entities or things. In other words, the temporary amalgamation of various parts of these basic constituents results in an individual something that is a compartmentalization of the basic fabric of being. While that may sound extremely complicated, it is simple if we assume that whatever forces and energies make up the universe are present in all things. This "basic fabric of being" looks different, depending on how it is organized.

To illustrate, bubbles in a stream are circumscribed compartments of air and water. Yet, for a time, they are individual bubbles, their uniqueness depending on the relationship and patterning of their components or substrates. These relationships, this patterning, formation, or organization are dependent on the phenomenon we will term *information*.

Information, as used in systems theories, is not just a message passed from one person to another. Information is contained within an object, such as a pencil, whether it is in use or not. Information is the power of organization, for, by it, the entity assumes the relationships that give it form and function (7). The information contained within the pencil is what gives it the properties of a pencil. All the information is coded and stored within the system *mind* that processes it. A plant differs from a rock because of the information (power of organization) its constituent parts receive and process. Information must have a matter/energy carrier and any matter/energy carrier contains information.

A Systems Approach All the various interacting coded information that makes up the universe is arranged in open systems. A *system* can be defined as a set of phenomena relating to and influencing each other (7). The system is recognizable as a whole even though the constituent phenomena may be replaced by similar phenomena (8). Any part of an automobile can be replaced by a similar part and we will still recognize it as an automobile.

The properties of a system are different from that of any of its components. The components of a system and their relationship may be viewed, as we have said, as coded information. In an open system, information is

Qualities of a system
1. Open
2. Constituant phenomenon replaced by like

continually flowing within the system and between the system and its environment. Information might be less fluid within a closed system but no one has as yet been able to find a closed system. So no matter what we study, we are studying the generation, movement, and storage of coded information among open systems.

As we have already stressed, *information* is a characteristic of organization, structure, and function. Information may also be defined as any influence that affects relationships within a system or between the system and its environment. Such influences may result in change or stability.

Basically, then, systems theories are concerned with the organization of matter and energy as determined and regulated by the flow of information and evidenced in a series of relationships and their interactions (7).

A running automobile is a functioning open system composed of several components or subsystems in a relationship that is regulated by information. The amount of gasoline taken into a cylinder of the engine mixed with air and combusted is regulated in part by the information transmitted to the engine by pressure on the accelerator and partly by information built into the system earlier in terms of such variables as carburetor size and cylinder volume.

A nonrunning automobile is also an open system, but its functions are different. What is the difference between the information being processed by the running car and the information being processed by the nonrunning car? Both have engines, both look like automobiles; but one runs and the other does not. The running vehicle is being influenced (receiving and processing information) so that its component parts relate in such a way as to function as a running car. The difference, then, between a running and a nonrunning car is dependent on information flow.

If we use a systems approach as one way of conceptualizing the universe, we might say that our entire universe can be appreciated as the interaction of coded information. This holds true whether we speak of the universe as interacting mass and energy or as resonating force fields. When we speak of forces, whether we denote them as positive or negative, centripetal or centrifugal, we are designating a type of coded information that has bearing on relationships.

Relationships Biased by Sensory Organs

In addressing dynamic relationships, we are always biased by our sensory organs. Our eyes, ears, organs of touch and smell are adjusted in such a way that the properties of many relationships give the impression of form. If the relationships are changing at speeds and magnitudes in which our sense organs can perceive motion we are aware of the process. All relationships are processes—slow or fast. Those with the time period outside our perceptive sensitivity have the property of form.

For example, the relationship of wind and water can be seen as waves. The relationship of wind and stone is outside our perceptive realm, and the stone, although interacting with the wind, appears to keep its form. We cannot see the oscillation of its components or the slow erosion that will change the rock. We *can* see the appearance and disappearance of the waves in the water. An example of a series of relationships too fast to be discerned by our sensory organs is a chair. The relationships among the molecules which make up the chair are moving much too rapidly for us to see the process we call a chair.

Since rapidly changing relationships are difficult to describe, we use words and concepts that imply form. To use another illustration, we may say, on seeing a twisting, flowing body of water, "It's a river." Subtly, we have concretized a fluid interaction of earth and water. It is similar to catching the river in a bucket. The water in the bucket was once part of the river but once in the bucket all relationships are changed and we can no longer call it a river.

Relationships as Entities

Whatever we arbitrarily or pragmatically denominate as the basic building blocks of being, the patterned relationships of these units are equally as important as the units themselves in determining the properties of anything that appears to exist. But most of our attention has been focused on the units rather than on the relationships and, until this century, the question of relationships was largely in the domain of metaphysics, religion, and the Eastern philosophies.

Why has it been so difficult for us to address the concept of relationships?

From childhood we learn to name things—first things different from us, then ourselves as different from things. A premium is placed on differentiating.

While we are learning to differentiate ourselves, we

are covertly sitting outside our environment. We believe we can be nonbiased observers. However, we are continually interacting with the environment we are observing. The very attitude of being outside the relationship we are observing distorts our point of view.

We may say, "I am observing a bean plant." It would be just as accurate to describe the effect that light waves reflected from a function called a bean plant is having on the chemical relationships in our central nervous system. The bean plant being observed is not a static absolute but a dynamic interaction of our organized information derived from our present and past experiences with bean plants. We share the environment with the bean plant and our observations are based on the alterations the bean plant makes on this environment by reflecting light or resisting pressure from our touch.

If our ears were tuned to the right frequencies, we would be able to hear the plant's living processes. All these stimuli (information) are compared with stored information (memory). We say, "That's a bean plant" because some other person said that particular experience was a bean plant.

We must remember that we are also changing the environment (for example, by breathing, affecting the lighting in the laboratory, touching the plant, producing air currents), so that the function of the bean plant is changed by our presence while we are making observations.

In a human–bean plant relationship, the distortions caused by assuming that the human observer is outside the environment may be of little consequence. However, it has far-reaching implications when the human observer is studying another human, as we shall illustrate in later chapters.

As our education progresses, we learn that things are composed of other things. We learn to accept that entities are composed of things that we cannot perceive with our unaided sense organs. A crystal of salt is composed of sodium and chloride atoms too small to be seen. This all follows a logical sequence until we encounter the concept that the whole might be different from the sum of its parts. This makes little sense to our linear logic until we adjust our conceptualizing machinery to consider the relationship among things as an entity in itself equally as important as the things. The crystalline property of a grain of salt is not the sodium and chloride atoms but their relationship in a space–time grid. The same atoms not in combination have different properties. Sodium is a solid quite unlike table salt, and chloride is a yellowish gas. In solutions of water, the relationship of sodium and chloride ions does not have the crystalline properties.

The difficulty in conceptualizing a relationship as a thing seems to arise in the changing rather than the static nature of this type of phenomenon. Static entities seem much more predictable even though they do not exist except in our thinking. As scientific study progresses, the number of things that we can consider as static absolutes becomes less and less until we slowly become suspicious that all perceivable things are illusions. Atoms, once thought to be basic building blocks, are now seen as complex harmonic relationships. Our concept of the world must, therefore, begin to change.

Influence of Nuclear Physics   Advances in the science of nuclear physics during the present century are helping us shift our concept of the world as being composed of discrete entities or mutable forms to a concept of the world as being composed of continually changing relationships, or fluid functions or processes, in open systems. So gradual has this shift been in our thinking that we have incorporated into our language phrases that carry much more import than we realize. We say "That's only relative" or "Relatively speaking" without being conscious that we are talking about fluid relationships rather than concrete absolutes.

Albert Einstein spent his lifetime developing theories of relativity. He utilized a system in which the distance between events is measured rather than the distance between objects, and space and time are encompassed together. It is a mathematically verifiable framework rooted not upon things or entities but upon relationships (4, 1).

Sir Arthur Stanley Eddington, a British astronomer famous for his studies of relativity and stellar evolution and the motions of the stars, wrote that the physical world is formed of building material composed of the mindstuff which is the "conglomeration of relations" (3). Thus, both Einstein and Eddington, among many others, emphasized relationships as the major focus for scientific and philosophical attention.

But to address relationships rather than the entities that are related remains a difficult task and, in many ways, resembles trying to catch the river in a bucket. It is much easier to say, "That's my car" than it is to say,

"That's a set of components interacting with one another in such a way as to make up a functioning open system." We cannot see, touch, or hear the relationships but we can see, touch, and hear the car concept. It is even more difficult to focus on relationships when we study living systems such as man.

The Environment

Not only must we focus on relationships, but we must consider the environment. Living systems must interact with the environment in order to maintain life. This means that any living system must be continually organizing information in order to stay alive. Once it stopped organizing information from its environment it would reach the relatively inert state of death.

Erwin Schrodinger, a Nobel prize-winning physicist (1933) famous for his work on quantum theory and wave mechanics, used the same terms for the phenomena of environmental interactions that are now frequently used by systems theorists. He called the organization of information *negative entropy,* and stated that the organism can stay alive only by pulling negative entropy or *negentropy* from its environment. *Positive entropy* is randomness or disorganization. *Maximum* entropy is the inert state, death (9).

As living systems, human beings must synchronize information from their external and internal environment for survival. In the human animal, survival is but one function. Another function is that of forming concepts such as those we have been discussing.

The Individual as a Series of Relationships

The next major step in our study of man, and a somewhat frightening one, is the realization that the perceivers of things, that is, we, the concept makers, are a series of harmonic relationships. Our bodies, with their millions of cells, each cell with its molecular arrangement, each molecule composed of atoms, and so on.

We have the illusion that the atoms composing our bodies are uniquely ours rather than having been used in many different relationships throughout evolution. The carbon atoms now in our bodies may have been involved in numerous plants, animals, and men before being incorporated in our transient form.

Life is a word used to describe a set of relationships or properties of relationships. Just as hardness is a property of the atomic relationships of a salt crystal, the relationship of certain atoms and molecules has properties that we term *life*. It is crucial to understand that the relationship is as important as the units that are related. Just as the atoms of a salt crystal may be replaced by similar atoms with no discernable difference in the properties we call crystalline, so, in living organisms, is there a constant replacement of atoms and molecules without changing the properties we call life. It seems true, however, that the new units need to be similar to those they replace in order to maintain predictable relationships. If the order of relationships is shifted, the crystal is changed and the living system is changed. The building blocks of crystals or of life, whether we conceptualize them as atoms or subatomic phenomena, are not sufficient to give the properties of life if not arranged in a given order. This order is dependent on coded information.

Living Systems   Living systems are similar to crystals in that the units composing both are related in a predictable order. However, in living systems, the ordering of relationships is more fluid and complex than those of familiar crystals such as table salt. The code of information that maintains predictable relationships in living systems is programmed for continual adjustment to maintain equilibrium or relative stability (homeostasis) in response to fluctuating data from the internal and external environments of the organism.

The code by which information is moved in a living system may be ionic, as in electrolyte balance, molecular as in DNA and RNA, hormonal as in thyroid–pituitary interaction, electrical as in neuronal transmission, or interorganismic by pheromones, gestures, cries or abstract speech. These codes are often interdependent, with one code system being translated into numerous code systems. *Biologic evolution* may be viewed as the acquisition by living matter of progressively more complex code systems with the potential for processing larger amounts of information.

This process began rather slowly if we consider the age of the earth to be about 5 billion years (5), with life beginning as a chemical chain reaction sometime during the earth's first 2000 million years (5). In its earliest stages, most of the coded information in living matter may be speculated to have been passed by ionic and molecular code systems until these codes reached sufficient intricacy to establish the interlocking relationships that we call a *cell*.

It has been postulated that the ability to organize and grow via self-regulating systems distinguishes living from non-living things. The study of crystal growth and organization, coupled with our beginning knowledge of crystalline viruses, makes this distinction seem somewhat arbitrary. With the advent of the cell, the properties of protoplasmic organization allow us to differentiate more easily between living and nonliving systems. We should keep in mind that this differentiation is a man-made working concept and not necessarily a break in the continuum of being.

During the past century, we have come to accept the cell as the basic building block of most living systems. In conceiving of a cell as a basic entity, we often slip into our habit of addressing it as though it were a static absolute—a thing. Continuing research in the field of cellular biology emphasizes that the cell is an enormously complex cybernetic interaction of coded data. It is an oversimplification to speak of cell wall, cytoplasm, and nucleus without some awareness of the interchange between DNA and RNA and their codes of nucleotides and amino acids. Each cell is a virtual library of coded data that continually shift and realign themselves in accord with the previously coded data. Again, we would like to focus on the concept we call the cell as a relationship among bits of coded information rather than as a thing. Any shift in the informational coding system results in a change in the balance between the internal and external milieu of the cell. It is through this process of mutation that living systems submit new organizations to the evolutionary contest. Certain shifts in the data-processing system of the cell may help it to adapt more productively to the data presented to it from its internal and external environment or it may result in the total breakdown of its data-processing machinery.

The changing programs of organization, continually biased by previously stored coded information, are relentlessly subjected to the test of survival. The evolution from subatomic elements via atoms, molecules, amino acids and nucleotides to the living cell and subsequent multicellular organisms is a continuum that we distort when we focus our attention on a part of the whole.

References   1. Bernstein, J. *Einstein.* New York: The Viking Press, 1973.

2. Bohr, Niels. Words spoken to Werner Heisenberg cited in Bronowski, J. *The Ascent of Man.* Boston: Little, Brown, 1973, p. 340.

3. Eddington, Sir A. Reality, causation, science and mysticism. In S. Commins and R. Linscott (Eds.), *Man and the universe, The philosophers of science.* New York: Washington Square Press, 1947. Pp. 412–470.

4. Einstein, A. The problem of space, ether, and the field in physics. In S. Commins and R. Linscott (Eds.), *Man and the universe, The philosophers of science.* New York: Washington Square Press, 1947. Pp. 471–484.

5. Hockett, C. *Man's place in nature.* New York: McGraw-Hill, 1973. Pp. 314 and 328.

6. Jeans, Sir J. Some problems of philosophy. In S. Commins and R. Linscott (Eds.), *Man and the universe, The philosophers of science.* New York: Washington Square Press, 1947. Pp. 361–410.

7. Miller, J. Living systems: Basic concepts. *Behavioral Science, 1965, 10,* 193–237.

8. Rapoport, A. General systems theory: A bridge between two cultures. Third Annual Ludwig von Bertalanffy Memorial Lecture. *Behavioral Science, 1976, 21,* 228–239.

9. Schrodinger, E. *What is life: And other scientific essays.* Garden City, New York: Doubleday, 1956. Pp. 70–71.

Suggested Readings

Bertalanffy, L. von. General systems theory and psychiatry—An overview. In W. Gray, F. Duhl, and N. Rizzo (Eds.), *General systems theory and psychiatry.* Boston: Little, Brown, 1969. Pp. 33–46.

Bronowski, J. *The ascent of man.* Boston: Little, Brown, 1973.

Calvin, M. Chemical evolution. *American Scientist, 1975, 63,* 169–177.

Darwin, C. *The origin of the species.* New York: Mentor Books, 1958.

Fuller, R. Buckminster, *Synergetics, explorations in the geometry of thinking.* New York: Macmillan, 1975.

Gray, W., and Rizzo, N. History and development of general systems theory. In W. Gray, F. Duhl, and N. Rizzo (Eds.), *General systems theory and psychiatry.* Boston: Little, Brown, 1969. Pp. 7–31.

Heisenberg, W. *Physics and philosophy, The revolution in modern science.* New York: Harper and Row, 1962.

Holden, A., and Singer, P. *Crystals and crystal growing.* Garden City, New York: Doubleday (Anchor Books), 1960.

Miller, J. *Living systems.* New York: McGraw-Hill, 1977.

Miller, J. General systems theory. In A. Freedman, H. Kaplan, and B. Sadock (Eds.), *Comprehensive textbook of psychiatry,* Vol. 1, 2nd ed. Baltimore: Williams and Wilkins, 1975. Pp. 75–88.

Murdy, W. Anthropocentrism: A modern version. *Science* 1975, *187*, 1168–1172.

Rapoport, A. Mathematical aspects of general systems analysis. *General Systems*, 1966, *11* (3).

Rapoport, A. Mathematics and Cybernetics. In S. Arieti (Ed.), *American handbook of psychiatry*, Vol. 1. New York: Basic Books, 1974. Pp. 1074–1094.

Shapley, H. *Beyond the observatory*. New York: Charles Scribner's Sons, 1967.

Sinnott, E. *Cell and psyche: The biology of purpose*. New York: Harper Torchbooks, 1961.

Sobel, D. Gravity and structural integration. In R. Ornstein (Ed.), *The nature of human consciousness, A book of readings*. New York: Viking, 1974. Pp. 397–407.

Whitehead, A. *Process and reality, An essay in cosmology*. New York: Free Press, 1969.

Wiener, N. *Cybernetics*. New York: Wiley, 1948.

Suggested Questions

1. What is the true object of scientific study?

2. Define the word *system* as used by systems theorists.

3. Define the word *information* as used by systems theorists.

4. With what are systems theories basically concerned?

5. Using systems theory, compare a running automobile with a nonrunning automobile.

6. How do our sensory organs bias us when we address dynamic relationships?

7. Discuss the difficulty in conceptualizing relationships.

8. How has the science of nuclear physics during the present century influenced our conceptual framework?

9. What is *negative entropy* and in what context do we use the term when referring to a living organism?

10. Give one definition of the word *life*.

11. What happens if the order of relationships is shifted in a living system?

12. How are living systems similar to crystals?

13. Using a systems approach, define biological evolution.

14. Why is it too simplistic to address the cell as though it were a static absolute—a thing?

2 Biological Evolution and Systems Theory

To put it briefly, we witness the event that existing order displays the power of maintaining itself and of producing orderly events.

Erwin Schrodinger, 1956(7)

The connection of the brain with mind seems to rest on the organization of the brain, and that organization is cell-organization.

Sir Charles Sherrington, 1940(8) p. 208

Evolution and Information Flow

With the evolution of the cell, life as an organization entered a new phase of data processing. The coded information contained in the protoplasm of a cell results in an exceedingly complex set of interacting systems mediated through atomic and molecular functions. Some of the functions of these systems regulated by coded information include metabolism, reproduction, irritability, and contractibility. These functions are associated with the cell's ability to respond to stimuli.

"Response to stimuli" implies that the cell receives and processes information that alters its internal relationships and the relationship between its internal and external environment. These alterations may affect other cells in the environment.

To illustrate, suppose we have several amoebas in a very small dish of water and we stimulate one amoeba with a tiny electrode. It may respond by expanding and contracting. Its movement causes movement in the water in the dish, and this fluid movement may stimulate the other amoebas. The movement of the rest of the amoebas in response to the information (or stimulus) applied by the electrode to one amoeba changes their relationships to their environment, thereby changing themselves *and* the environment. Their motion will, in turn, affect the amoeba we first stimulated. We now have a dynamic interacting system of stimuli causing response and response creating stimuli in a *feedback loop*.

To extrapolate, an alteration in one cell that results in information being submitted to another cell allows the potential for intercellular communication. This capability for data sharing was of crucial importance as cells began to live in close proximity to one another. With the exchange of information among cellular units, colonies of cells enhanced their chance of survival.

Consider again the dish of amoebas. The amoeba we stimulated with the electrode indirectly, through its movement, initiated movement in the other amoebas so that it would be more difficult to touch them with the electrode.

Information exchange catalyzed increasing dependency among cells living in colonies. These colonies were originally composed of cells that were more or less identical. By the process of mutation (alterations in internal organization), some of the cells began to differ from their neighbors. These specialized cells survived if they enhanced the data-processing efficiency of the colony. Some cells evolved that were more efficient at metabolic processes, others at reproduction, and still others that specialized in receiving and responding to stimuli. The sharing of information throughout the colony allowed its data processing system to be different from that which occurred in any single cell.

The relationship of a colony of interdependent specialized cells is called a *multicellular organism,* the survival of which is again dependent on the effectiveness of data processing.

The evolution of multicellular organisms, beginning perhaps 2 billion years ago with the appearance of multicellular filaments (5), resulted in and from more complex and adaptable inter- and intraorganismic coding of information. As evolution continued, cells in the multicellular complex became increasingly specialized. Those cells with an augmented response to stimuli differentiated into receptor and effector cells. The receptor cells received data from the outside or inside environment of the organism and arranged it into codes that could be used by the effector cells, whose information coding system resulted in organismic response. This organismic response now differs from the response of any individual cell within the open system.

Such an organization is a primitive neuromechanism, a mechanism still present in the aquatic coelenterates (for example, the hydra, jellyfish, and anemone), which have receptor and effector cells arranged throughout the organism in a neural net.

Centralization   With increasing organization of the multicellular organisms under the pressure of natural selection, those cells which specialized in the processing of new data, that is, the precursors of neurons, tended to align themselves in groups, or ganglia, a process known as *centralization*. From these aggregates of neural cells came the beginning of complex reflex arcs, whereby stimuli are received by sensitive cells and relayed through association cells, which further process the data and send the coded information to effector cells, which adjust the animal's relationship to its environment.

The process by which neural tissue progressed from a ganglion to a neural tube and the subsequent cephalization (development of a centralized brain) is described in textbooks of zoology and neuroanatomy (11, 12). As we study the phylogenetic development of central nervous systems, especially the human brain, we become aware of the large number of subsystems of which it is composed. Some of these subsystems are newer than others, having evolved by mutation much later.

Cybernetic Quality   During the evolution of the human central nervous sys-
of All Systems   tem, the primitive organ which resembled a toti potential nerve net or reticular formation underwent wave after wave of specialization in the sensory–motor and association functions. Each new specialized subsystem added a dimension to the information processing paradigm.

As neuronal systems specialized in sensory–motor and association activity, a central core system evolved to regulate the state of activity of other subsystems in the brain. This activating system controls the state of arousal of an organism, and thereby influences its information processing and subsequent behaviors, or observable actions. The work of Moruzzi and Magoun has been a major contribution to our appreciation of a central activating system (6).

The amount of information processed, the coding of data and its storage, is continually influenced by the individual's state of arousal. Conversely, the state of arousal is influenced by the quantity and quality of information passing through and relayed back to the activating system. The behavioral readout of the individual is colored by systems concerned with emotion. These systems may be thought of as phylogenetically evolved elaborations of the energizing or activating systems, and they modulate the intensity and quality of response to information from internal and external sources.

Figure 2.1 is a simplified diagram, using a systems approach of the interaction among neural systems and between these systems and the environment. The figure illustrates the cybernetic (feedback) activity of the systems. Sensory data influence the state of arousal and emotional tone within the system. Motor activity in response to sensory, arousal, and emotional information shifts the individual's relationship to its environment, thereby altering the energies applied to the sensory system. Since all these systems are interdependent and over-

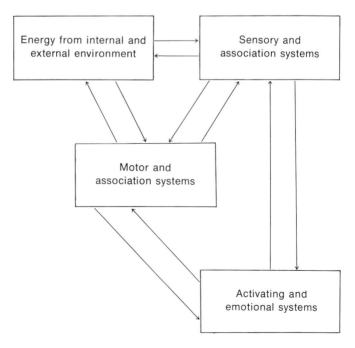

FIGURE 2.1
Neural system–
environment
interactions.

lapping, it is a distortion to consider them as discrete closed systems.

Tendency to Concretize Systems

There has been a tendency for scientific investigation to focus on the specific function of each of these collaborating subsystems whether it be the not-so-simple reflex arc or other subsystems which have been delineated and given such names as the reticular system, hypothalamic system, thalamic system, limbic system, pyramidal system, and extrapyramidal system. Although this type of investigation has led to advances in our understanding of the arrangements within the central nervous system it may inadvertently have led us to concretize our concept of the central nervous system. We may begin to think of each subsystem as separate and unique, working independently of other subsystems. This way of thinking about the central nervous system has been reinforced by the information obtained from neuropathology. Lesions in one area of the central nervous system may produce different effects from lesions in another area. For example, destruction of a small portion of the human neocortex in the dominant cerebral hemisphere has a devastating effect on an individual's ability to communicate. A lesion of the same size and position (near the junction of the parietal and occipital lobes) in the nondominant hemisphere might have less dramatic effect.

The delineation or differentiation of various subsystems within the central nervous system is a useful working concept and helps us increase our knowledge of human behavior if we remember that isolation of any part of a fluid open system is a distortion.

We are becoming more aware not only of the anatomical complexity of the central nervous system but also of the elaborate enzyme systems and the large numbers of chemical substances involved in the transmission, coding, and storing of information. This mode of study is vital to the fields of neural and behavioral sciences, but is outside the scope of this book.

Relationship of All Cells and Systems in the Central Nervous System

As we consider the central nervous system and its various subsystems, we are really addressing a large colony of specialized cells of various types. These cells within the central nervous system are directly or indirectly related. To emphasize this point, let us imagine each cell of the human nervous system dissected out of its relationship with other cells and maintained alive in a culture medium. Although to do this would be technically impossible, all the cellular elements of the central nervous system might be sustained for a period of time in artificial media.

As we surveyed our millions of culture dishes, each containing a living cell pulsating in its media, we would be struck by the similarity between these tiny living systems and their distant cousin, the amoeba. Having accomplished this Herculean task, we might pose the question, "How do we pick the cell responsible for human thought?" Although this hypothetical situation might seem somewhat absurd, it again emphasizes that relationships and the organization of relationships of units are as important as the units themselves. The function of the relationships of the cells of the brain is quantitatively and qualitatively different from the function of any given cell.

The Human Mind as a Continuum of Related Information

Although we can discuss the relationships that make up the brain, it is exceedingly difficult to define what it is we are looking for when we talk about the "mind." So far, we have been discussing a large colony of specialized cells of various types, which we have called the "brain." Where is the "mind," which is doing the thinking and forming the concepts? Can we localize the mind?

In his book, *Man on His Nature*, Sherrington has beautifully demonstrated the futility of attempting to localize the human mind in a delineated neural constellation (8). This impasse has also been eloquently addressed by Eddington in his essay, "Reality, Causation, Science and Mysticism" from his book *The Nature of the Physical World* (3).

Research in brain–mind liaison done by Levy, Sperry, Eccles, and others, although meticulous in its organization and revealing in its description of various anatomical functions, leaves us with the uncomfortable conclusion that the relationship of the human mind to specific areas in the brain can most accurately be described at present as a subject of speculation (2).

As a broad definition, we may postulate that the *mind* is a continuum of related information, a relationship that encompasses all the data processed within the individual, including data stored during billions of light years of inorganic evolution and eons of biologic evolution, that is, data stored in chromosomes as well as all the data processed from the experiences the individual has shared with others throughout the transient period we call a lifetime.

Our most remarkable biologic function is our behavior as a collectivity of information exchange. The lives of humans are spent in an information-exchange system, so that it appears that all human minds behave together as one open interacting system of thought (10).

This definition indicates the interrelationship of information stored in humanity with all the information in our solar system and perhaps the universe. The human mind is then conceptualized as an arbitrary delineation in the information continuum. This definition incorporates Sinnott's thesis that biologic organization is fundamentally the same as the mind (9) and also allows philosophic speculations concerning the mind or will permeating the universe. Although these speculations are intriguing and help to expand our often too anthropocentric perspectives, they shift our endeavors into the realm of metaphysics, where the fabric of logic becomes somewhat frayed.

We must create our own images when we describe the invisible world. Our destiny is that we acquire knowledge. However, there can be no certainty in that knowledge. Modern physics, especially that interpretation put forth by Werner Heisenberg in the principle of uncertainty suggests that all information is limited. So it must be with the mind—its description can never be total and its boundaries can never be localized (1).

The term *mind* with all its implications seems too encompassing to utilize in a working model for students of human behavior. How, then, can we address the phenomena of human consciousness and thought?

The Bimodal System of Data Processing

If we return to the cell or neuron as a starting point, we can empirically divide its data-processing activity into two overlapping modes, the continuous and the interrupted. Afferent signals from a given stimulus travel along dendrites (nerve fibers conducting toward the cell bodies) in interrupted bursts. They arrive at the cell bodies where they are summated, attenuated, or digested in a continuous fashion. If the information processed within a cell reaches a critical level, the cell relays the coded information to other cells through interrupted bursts of activity via its axon (a nerve fiber conducting away from the cell body). For a more detailed description of these processes, refer to John C. Eccles' book, *The Understanding of the Brain* (2).

We will term the continuous mode of information coding *analogical* and the interrupted mode, *digital*. This model is discussed at some length by Ralph Gerard, Norbert Wiener, and others in the *Transactions of the Seventh Conference on Cybernetics* edited by Heinz von Foerster (4).

We will develop as our working hypothesis that the bimodal data-processing model can be productively applied to the activity of the entire constellation of cells comprising the central nervous system. This is a pragmatic model that allows us to develop analogies useful in understanding human behavior.

References

1. Bronowski, J. *The ascent of man.* Boston: Little, Brown, 1973.

2. Eccles, J. *The understanding of the brain.* New York: McGraw-Hill, 1973.

3. Eddington, Sir A. Reality, causation, science and mysticism. In S. Commins and R. Linscott (Eds.), *Man and the universe, The philosophers of science.* New York: Washington Square Press, 1947. Pp. 412–470.

4. Foerster, H. von (Ed.). *Cybernetics: Circular causal and feedback mechanisms in biological and social systems,* Transactions of the Seventh Conference, March 23–24, 1950, New York. Caldwell, New Jersey: Josiah Macy, Jr. Foundation, Progress Associates, 1951.

5. Hockett, C. *Man's place in nature.* New York: McGraw-Hill, 1973.

6. Magoun, H. *The waking brain,* 2nd ed. Springfield, Illinois: Charles C Thomas, 1963.

7. Schrodinger, E. *What is life and other scientific essays.* Garden City, New York: Doubleday, 1956, p. 75.

8. Sherrington, Sir C. *Man on his nature.* London: Cambridge University Press, 1940.

9. Sinnott, E. *Cell and psyche: The biology of purpose.* New York: Harper Torchbooks, 1961.

10. Thomas, L. *The lives of a cell: Notes of a biology watcher.* New York: Viking, 1974.

11. Truex, R., and Carpenter, M. *Human neuroanatomy.* Baltimore: Williams and Wilkins, 1969.

12. Willis, W., Jr., and Grossman, R. *Medical neurobiology.* Saint Louis: C. V. Mosby, 1973.

Suggested Readings

Bergson, H. The evolution of life. In S. Commins and R. Linscott (Eds.). *Man and the universe, The philosophers of science*. New York: Washington Square Press, 1947. Pp. 277–297.

Edwards, P. (Ed.). *The nature of man*. New York: Macmillan, 1968.

Fromm, E., and Xirau, R. *The nature of man*. New York: Macmillan, 1971.

Huxley, J. *Evolution in action*. New York: Mentor Books, 1957.

Lorenz, K. Analogy as a source of knowledge, *Science*, 1974, *185*, 229–234.

Lowenberg, B. (Ed.). *Charles Darwin: Evolution and natural selection*. Boston: Beacon Press, 1959.

Suggested Questions

1. Describe what is meant by the phrase "response to stimuli," with reference to a cell.

2. Describe how the alteration in one cell may influence another cell.

3. List one factor that may allow a specialized cell to survive.

4. What is centralization?

5. Discuss the functions of systems associated with emotion.

6. Discuss the pros and cons of studying isolated subsystems within the central nervous system.

7. How is the function of the relationships of the cells of the brain different from the function of any given cell?

8. Give a broad definition of the concept "mind."

9. Discuss the difficulty of attempting to localize the boundaries of the mind.

10. What is our most remarkable biological function?

11. Discuss information processing of a nerve cell using the analog and digital model.

3 Bimodal Coding

There must be something unique about man because otherwise, evidently, the ducks would be lecturing about Konrad Lorenz, and the rats would be writing papers about B. F. Skinner.

Jacob Bronowski, 1973(3)

Cybernetic Movement of Information

Like the individual neuron, the entire central nervous system responds to stimuli. Specialized receptor organs respond to information presented to them by shifting patterns of light waves, sound waves, pressure, and molecular concentration. These responses are translated into codes (chemical and electrical), which are transmitted to sensory and association centers where the information is assimilated, translated to other codes, stored, and often transmitted again to other organs. If these coded messages are relayed to effector organs, the information may result in muscle contraction or glandular secretion, which alter the organism's internal or external relationships. This alteration results in a new series of afferent stimuli relayed back to the central nervous system with subsequent readjustment. In this cybernetic (feedback) movement of information, the data may be coded and recoded many times.

For example, a man starts across a street. Light waves reflected from an oncoming car enter his eye, setting up chemical and electrical charges. These charges are codes of information that are transmitted to his brain, where they undergo further electrical and chemical changes (recoding of information). This information is compared with information stored from previous experiences so that the man becomes aware of a change in his environment, called a car, which is moving toward him.

These data are also processed by other brain systems, including those associated with the man's state of arousal, emotion, and his motor activity, which activate his muscle tissue and he jumps back. The movement of his muscles and the pressure of the cement sidewalk send messages back to the brain concerning his posture and position. These messages are coded and organized by the brain, resulting in further messages to various muscles in his limbs and body so that he regains his balance on the curb and focuses his eyes on the passing car. This is an oversimplification, since each system within a person's body interacts with all other systems by feedback loops (cybernetically). Every system in the man's body is involved in this one little jump!

Division of Coding Activity of the Central Nervous System

As we stated at the closing of the last chapter, in order to develop a working concept, we will divide the coding activity of the central nervous system into two major categories, although the exact boundary between these categories is somewhat arbitrary. In the first category—the *analogic system*—data are integrated continuously into an operational gestalt, or maplike picture, perhaps similar to a hologram. In the second category—the *digital system*, data are processed into individual units. The information is interrupted or chopped into segments, with each segment or unit containing data.

At this point you may ask, "Why should we divide information processing into two categories?" It does seem rather complicated but, in the following chapters, we will need this concept to help us better understand the human verbal and nonverbal communication process. It will seem less complicated as we continue to elaborate.

A number of investigators have utilized a bimodal model of data processing as a working analogy in attempting to better conceptualize human behavior as illustrated in Table 1, adapted from Bogen (2). It is of note that Bateson and Jackson, Ruesch and Kees, and Pribram have also utilized the terms *analog* and *digital*.

The digital and analogic data-processing operations form a continuum so that it is difficult to distinguish exactly where the hologram-like picture of the analog becomes segmentalized into the units of the digital. There is a continual conversion of the code from digital to analog to digital, etc., so that at any given time, we may

Table 1 Bimodal Models of Data Processing

Investigator	Interrupted or digital	Continuous or analog
Freud	Secondary process	Primary process
Pavlov	Second Signaling	First signaling
W. James	Differential	Existential
Pribram	Digital	Analogic
J. Z. Young	Abstract	Maplike
Bateson and Jackson	Digital	Analogic
Reusch	Digital or discursive	Analogic or eidetic
Goldstein	Abstract	Concrete
Head	Symbolic or systematic	Perceptual or nonverbal
Wilder	Numerical	Geometric
Price	Analytic or reductionist	Synthetic or concrete
C. S. Smith	Atomistic	Gross
Levi-Strauss	Positive	Mythic
Bruner	Rational	Metaphoric
Hobbes	Directed	Free or unordered
Schenov (Luria)	Successive	Simultaneous

refer to the relationship between these codes as the analog-to-digital ratio.

This hypothetical division of information coding into analog and digital is a pragmatic working concept, or analogy, and not a scientifically proven fact. Although there may be some superficial similarity, we do not mean to imply that the terms analog and digital carry the same definition as when they are used in computer terminology (1,7). The bimodal analog and digital model for data processing may be used to conceptualize the information-coding activity in any living system. In the human, with an enlarged central nervous system, these data-processing paradigms have evolved in complexity and refinement to an almost qualitative difference from those of other species.

Elaborate Digital Format in Man

The most remarkable difference occurring in the brain of the human animal as compared to the brains of other animals appears to be the elaboration of the digital format whereby perception, that is, patterns of information, is unitized or digitalized more efficiently than in any other central nervous system. This segmentalization, or unitization, of data allows man to pair or couple these units or digits with sounds, gestures, and designs to form signs. A sign may now represent one of these digitalized units of information (12).

Even though we seem more efficient in sign making than other mammals, there is good evidence that many animals are capable of similar activity on a limited scale. The property that appears to differentiate the human is the ability to condense the information in these digital units so that we enter the second signal system, symbolization, or the system of abstractions where a vocal sound, gesture, or some structure represents a great deal of compressed and associated information in each unit or symbol (1).

By this latter process, we increased the complexity and efficiency of our intraspecies communication. We developed language. The second signal system—language—provided a means of coding information that facilitated the differentiation of various elements of the environment. More importantly, it allowed us to differentiate ourselves from our environment via self-conceptualization. This property not only helps us communicate more effectively with others via spoken and written words, but also permits a type of data processing that can plot perceptions effectively on a space–time grid, allowing a logical sequence or ordering of experiential phenomena, and, thereby, the ability to predict future data.

Attempts to Localize Central Nervous System Functions

Researchers have been attempting to localize the language functions of the central nervous system or at least to delineate certain areas of the brain that are most associated with these phenomena. The works of Sperry, Gardner, Ornstein, Fischer, and Young are extremely provocative. There is some indication that each of the two cerebral hemispheres of the adult human have specialized. The nondominant hemisphere seems mostly involved in the analogic or topographic programming of data, with the digital operation developing mostly in the dominant hemisphere (5).

The left hemisphere, which is considered to be the dominant one in most right-handed people and in two-thirds of the left-handed people, is involved in arithmetic, writing, speech, and language. It is the field-articulating hemisphere that functionally digitalizes, analyzes, differentiates, and perceives sequences. The right, or nondominant, hemisphere is concerned with analog-type functions such as synthesizing (i.e., constructing the total picture) and processing nonverbal information. It is implicated in such activities as music, intuition, and imagery (6).

Attempts to localize anatomical mechanisms inside the central nervous system by such structuralists as Chomsky, Piaget, Levi-Strauss, and Jakobson may be destined to fail because of the close connection of the functions discovered to the interaction of neural mechanisms. However, structuralists are encouraged by the indications that, in brain-damaged individuals, the capacity for logic and linguistic creativity collapses along predictable lines (8). Studies on aphasia (inability to speak) certainly add credence to this hypothesis (9).

Nevertheless, the flexibility of the brains of children raises many questions about the hows and whys of this type of localization (10). Young children who have the left hemisphere surgically removed may learn to speak with the remaining right hemisphere.

For the purposes of this presentation, we will address the analogic and digital coding of data as functions without attempting to localize them to specific anatomical structures within the human brain.

Perception of Stimuli and the Bimodal Model

Let us now apply our bimodal data-processing model to the information flow that occurs in our perception of stimuli.

Perception of a given stimulus is dependent on contrasts in the perceiver's environment, which result in variation or modulation of the electromagnetic, chemical, or mechanical energy impinging on the sensory organs. We perceive a picture because the light reflected from certain parts is different from the light reflected from other parts. Without the differences and contrasts we would describe the paper as blank. These differences and contrasts allow our analogic paradigm for coding data to form a topographic maplike code of information proportional to the gradients of energy applied to the receptor organs. The contrasts or differences are magnified when the data are processed in the digital operation. The continuum, or gradual shifting between differential energies is interrupted. This is similar to breaking a curve or waveform into multiple points. The larger the number of points, the more accurately the curve is coded. Interrupting the continuous curve into discontinuous separate units always produces distortion.

For the sake of analogy, let us return to the example of a picture, say that of a dog. Our visual sense organ can analogically code a similar picture in memory storage systems. As we attempt to convert this analogic operation into the digital units coupled with words, we say, "It's the picture of a dog." Then we attempt to refine our abstraction by adding more digital points—we describe it as a large, brown, shaggy dog. The more points, the more accurate the code and yet, the breaking of the perception into units distorts, so that it would be difficult for another individual to take all these units or words and construct a picture exactly like the original without having seen the original.

Despite the distortion, the compression of data into communication units called signs and symbols makes for an efficient code of exchanging information and cueing memory patterns. We do not have to carry our dog or its picture to communicate to our neighbors about our pet. We substitute signs and symbols. We convert the gestalt of analogically coded information concerning our dog into a few specific units of the digital system.

Analog-to-Digital Ratio

The facility for analog-to-digital conversion and the digital-to-digital association of coded information may be called *intellect* or *intelligence*. This property of central nervous activity is dependent on many factors. At any given time, the analog-to-digital ratio is contingent on the individual's state of arousal and emotional tone.

Hypoarousal and hyperarousal shift the ratio toward the analogical side. When we become drowsy or fall asleep we have more difficulty in converting the stimuli presented to us into a logical sequence or words. Similarly, when we become extremely excited or panicked, our words fail us.

Research data indicate that there is a progressive increase in activity of the right hemisphere, which is concerned with the symbolic, visuospatial, and nonverbal functions, during hyperarousal and hypoarousal. It is believed that when we are neither hypo- nor hyperaroused (for example, during most of our regular activities) we utilize our major and minor hemispheres as the task demands. In other words, we may freely choose to move from the cognitive or dominant (Aristotelian major) hemisphere to the symbolic, visuospatial, nondominant (Platonic minor) hemisphere, or conversely, when desirable (6).

Figures 3.1 and 3.2 are diagrammatic representations of information flow among the open systems that we designate as human. Systems are labeled by function rather than by anatomical designation. The self-system will be explained in a later chapter.

The analog-to-digital ratio is dependent not only on the equipment we inherit for the analog-to-digital (A–D) conversion, but on our learning experiences. An environment rich in digitally coded information allows the development of a much broader base for digital operation than an environment with minimal digital input.

Let us emphasize again that information processing involves continual harmonious interaction of all systems within the human body. However, since this book is composed of written words, we are utilizing a digital mode of information exchange which distorts by differentiating. This distortion will be continually evident as we focus more on the central nervous system and its

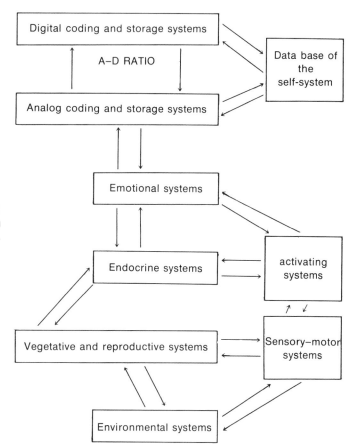

FIGURE 3.1
Information flow among
human open systems.

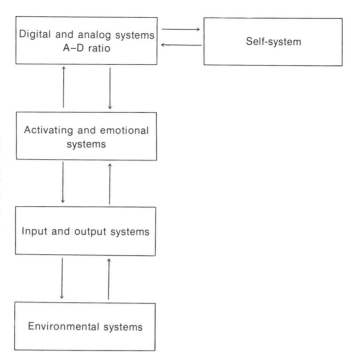

FIGURE 3.2
Figure 3.1 can be further
subdivided and assigned
to anatomical regions or
it can be amalgamated
into larger open systems
as here.

data-processing activity than on other systems with which it is continually and openly interacting.

It is important to note that the endocrine system, the cardiovascular system, the reproductive system, the renal system, the gastrointestinal system, the respiratory system, and all other systems and subsystems within the body are involved in producing, sustaining, and responding to states of arousal, emotions, and to the maintenance of the central nervous system. The analog-to-digital ratio of data processing within the central nervous system is dependent on the interactions of its entire internal and external environment.

Efficiency of Analog-to-Digital Conversion

The analog-to-digital conversion, that is, the compression of information into units and the coupling of these units with words we call language adds to our efficiency by (a) facilitating communication, and (b) providing a method for coding the data stored in our memory banks.

Although much data are continually stored in the analogic type of memory, it is sometimes more difficult to cue memories that consist of sensory imagery and other gestalts than those memories coded in symbols or words. For example, a certain odor may evoke a gestalt memory including a very complex set of associated data about persons, places, and times when a similar stimulus was present. This is a less efficient cue than the use of a word designating an object or person, by which we can selectively stimulate our memory banks to focus on a specific set of data. Increased capability in retrieval of memory data via this cueing mechanism is associated with our intricate social networks and technologic achievements that have enhanced our ability to survive in a wide range of environments.

Undoubtedly, one of the most far-reaching implications of the digital coding system, especially when this code is coupled with words that have been standardized in a social unit, is the efficiency in exchanging data among individuals. By the digital operation, standardized units can be coupled, aligned, arranged, and rearranged in an infinite number of sequences. Were these sequences random, processing of data, its storage and retrieval, would be chaotic and perhaps of little survival value. The human central nervous system has evolved a fairly standard format for plotting digitalized data. This format is analogous to Chomsky's term "syntax" (4). According to Chomsky, the human mind is naturally logical and rational, and one of its functions is a capacity for linguistics. Experience or environment are not of paramount significance, for the human brain has innate capacity for ideas. There are series of universal rules in the structure of the human brain which allow the acquisition of language (8).

The precision of ordering and coupling of units with words may differ among individuals and social groups. Yet, the genetically evolved pattern or ordering of digital data allows translation of coded information from one language to another. So far as we know, all recorded human language is translatable into a code we can understand today. However, the symbols used to represent the data compressed into digital units differ widely from culture to culture, often making translation difficult (11).

This linear ordering of digital data is associated with the phenomenon termed *linear logic*.

Coded information about one event in time and space is associated with similar data from a subsequent event, and, should this sequence recur, the data are often said to show a cause-and-effect relationship. This type of data processing allows us to extrapolate from previous data to anticipated data much more efficiently than other animals with less elaborate digital operations.

The digital operation not only enhances differentiation of objects perceived but also the differentiation of the perceiver from the perceived. Thus, the digital operation is associated with the subject–object dichotomy and linear logic—two phenomena of enormous importance in social evolution.

By this data-processing paradigm, we could more efficiently conceptualize ourselves and a cause-and-effect relationship among events in our environment. By coupling these two phenomena, we could code a relationship between our activities and our environment. From experiences, we were able to anticipate the effect our activities might have on future relationships. The survival value of this empirical system of coding digital data as a problem-solving device outweighed the distortions that are now becoming apparent.

References

1. Bateson, G. *Steps to an ecology of mind.* New York: Ballantine Books, 1972.

2. Bogen, J. The other side of the brain: An appositional mind. In R. Ornstein (Ed.), *The nature of human consciousness, A book of readings.* New York: Viking, 1974. Pp. 101–125.

3. Bronowski, J. *The ascent of man.* Boston: Little, Brown, 1973, p. 412.

4. Chomsky, N. *Language and mind.* New York: Harcourt Brace Jovanovich, 1972.

5. Dimond, S., and Beaumont, J. *Hemisphere function in the human brain.* New York: Wiley, 1974.

6. Fischer, R. Hallucinations can reveal creative imagination. *Fields within fields,* 1974, No. *11,* 29–31.

7. Foerster, H. von (Ed.). *Cybernetics: Circular causal and feedback mechanisms in biological and social systems,* Transactions of the Seventh Conference, March 23–24, 1950, New York. Caldwell, New Jersey: Josiah Macy, Jr. Foundation, Progress Associates, 1951.

8. Gardner, H. *The quest for mind.* New York: Random House (Vintage), 1974.

9. Gardner, H. *The shattered mind: The person after brain damage.* New York: Alfred A. Knopf, 1975.

10. Gazzaniga, M. The split brain in man. In R. Ornstein (Ed.), *The nature of human consciousness, A book of readings.* New York: Viking, 1974. Pp. 87–100.

11. Lee, D. Codifications of reality, lineal and non-lineal. In R. Ornstein (Ed.), *The nature of human consciousness, A book of readings.* New York: Viking, 1974. Pp. 128–142.

12. White, L. The symbol: The origin and basis of human behavior. In J. Jennings and E. Hoebel (Eds.), *Readings in anthropology,* 3rd ed. New York: McGraw-Hill, 1972. Pp. 315–321.

Suggested Readings

Chomsky, N. Linguistic contributions to the study of mind: Future. In Parveen Adams (Ed.), *Language in thinking.* Hammondsport, England: Penguin Books, 1972.

Deikman, A. Bimodal consciousness. In R. Ornstein (Ed.), *The nature of human consciousness, A book of readings.* New York: Viking, 1974. Pp. 67–86.

Eccles, J. *The understanding of the brain.* New York: McGraw-Hill, 1973.

Fischer, R. On separateness and oneness. *Confinia Psychiatrica,* 1972, *15,* 165–194.

Ornstein, R. *The psychology of consciousness.* New York: Viking, 1972.

Sperry, R. Cerebral dominance in perception. In F. Young and D. Lindsley (Eds.), *Early experience in visual information processing in perceptual and reading disorders.* Washington, D.C.: National Academy of Sciences, 1970.

Whitehead, A. *Science and the modern world.* New York: Free Press, 1967.

Young, J. *A model of the brain.* Oxford: Clarendon Press, 1960.

Suggested Questions

1. Give an example of the cybernetic (feedback) movement of information among the interacting systems of an individual.

2. Discuss the analog and digital coding paradigms.

3. What appears to be the most remarkable difference between the human brain and the brains of other animals?

4. What advantages has the development of language given man?

5. Contrast the apparent functions of the right and left hemispheres of the human brain.

6. Discuss the advantage of being able to compress data into communication units called signs and symbols.

7. Give one definition of intellect or intelligence.

8. Discuss how emotion affects the analog to digital (A–D) ratio.

9. On what is the A–D ratio dependent?

10. State two ways in which A–D conversion adds to our efficiency.

11. With what two phenomena in social evolution is the digital operation of man associated? Elaborate on each.

4 Digital Coding and the Acquisition of Language

At the crudest level of description, we may say that a language associates sound and meaning in a particular way; to have command of a language is to be able, in principle, to understand what is said and to produce a signal with an intended semantic interpretation.

Noam Chomsky, 1972(2) p. 115

Finally, we found that man does not develop language if he grows up among animals or in isolation. Language is acquired by the human being born into a linguistic community

Roger Brown, 1958(1) p. 193

Development of Human Symbolic Operations

In the previous chapter we addressed the analogic and digital modes of data processing, which are seen throughout all living systems, placing the human animal on a continuum with other species. In this chapter we will address the process by which the digital operation of the person is coupled with words. These words may be divided into two classes—*signs* and *symbols*.

Linguists and anthropologists often emphasize the difference between signs and symbols as codes for the movement of information. Many believe that signs and symbols are qualitatively different modes of communication. However, there is still some question as to whether this difference is quantitative rather than qualitative, a matter of degree rather than of kind.

In a series of differently shaped objects, one can learn to choose a cross from a circle. In this context, the word *cross* is a sign for a particular form or shape. In the sentence, *We all have our cross to bear,* the same word carries a great deal more abstract information, particularly in certain social situations, and therefore becomes a symbol. Both phenomena are readouts of the digital operation. Both contain compressed data that has been unitized or "chopped" from the analogic information-coding system.

In human communication, the same word, gesture, or design may be used as a sign or a symbol. The difference between signs and symbols, then, becomes a matter of the quantity of coded information in the unit, word, or design with the sign being more stimulus locked and the symbol requiring social validation for complete comprehension of its coded information. The human uses both of these digital operations.

Nonhuman Communication   Most higher animals can be taught rather complicated sign language, even using words as signs. Complex sign language very nearly approaching symbolic communication has been observed in some of the social insects. This has been described by Karl von Frisch (1945) in his studies of the waggle dance of the bee. "Symbolism occurs in the form of the ritualized straight run" (17). He indicated that "the communicator can generate new messages" (17) by means of what he terms symbolism and he postulates that the bee's target is "spoken of" in abstract fashion since it is "an object removed in time and space" (17). It has been argued that this type of communication lacks the abstraction of symbolism since the straight run is merely a reenactment of the flight the bee will take.

The format for this code might be considered analogic in nature since the dance is similar to drawing a map as opposed to the more abstract digital form of communication that we find in human language where directions are compressed into words.

Jane Goodall indicates that chimpanzees have a wide range of calls, each call being "fairly reliably associated with some specific emotion—a scream usually signifies fear, a bark, aggression, and so on. This means that the chimpanzee is able to communicate reasonably specific information about his feelings and his environment through the use of calls alone [15, p. 10]." She does not believe that these calls are specifically analogous to human language.

A number of birds have been trained to imitate human

language, but there is no good indication that the birds are able to communicate abstractly through this medium.

Chomsky indicates that the more profitable approach to the study of the comparison of human and other animal communication would be to define the structure of language rather than discussing the reasons for which it is used. He postulates that the language of the human animal is different from that of other animals because of the way it is organized. His theories seem to emphasize the relationship among units of information rather than the information contained in each unit (3).

Development of Linguistic Skills in Children

The study of the process by which children move from sign language to symbolic communication has been enormously advanced by the work of Vygotsky, Stanislavsky, Piaget, Langer, and others. They indicate that speech begins first as an external phenomenon. The child practices vocalizing words, naming objects, and making sounds that can be validated by others before linguistic communication is internalized and synchronized with his own digital operation.

During the transition between external speech and the synchronization of speech with *intrapsychic functions* children use a type of expression termed *egocentric speech*. They are apparently attempting to coordinate their internal analog and digital programming activities with perceptions arising from their external world, including communications from others. During this operation the intrapsychic activities or thoughts (analog and digital operations) are made to harmonize with linguistic output. In this operation there is a movement from less structured totipotential expressions to more standardized sets of linguistic symbols that are more likely to receive social validation. For example, a child may make gutteral sounds and wave his arms to imply a need. The mother may have to make several attempts to satisfy this need before appreciating that the child is thirsty. When the child masters the word "water", this simplifies the information exchange. Not only do children have to synchronize their abstract speech with their thought processes, but they must also coordinate the readout so they are understood by the people around them. Chomsky's work on the development of syntax, Shannon's paper on mathematical aspects of language, and Wierner's theories on cybernetics and communication help us appreciate the complexity of these feedback systems.

Studies on deaf-mute children indicate that the digital processing of data can be coupled with visual phenomena in place of the auditory cues of verbal language. This coupling can be accomplished with hand language and written words. Helen Keller's accomplishments indicate that the digital process might be independent of sight and hearing.

Humans are conditioned to utilize the semantic and phonetic format of their social systems, which influences the subsequent digital operation of the brain. As children learn or are conditioned to interlock their digital operation with the signs and symbols of their social systems and to couple this with their motor systems so that they are able to reproduce similar signs and symbols, they enter the world of symbolic communication, which is quantitatively different from any other form of animal communication of which we are presently aware.

Vygotsky has postulated the occurrence of internal speech (endosophy) that is not paired with words (16). This suggests that the digital operation precedes or is independent of social learning. Chomsky speaks of a universal grammar and theorizes that syntax and semantics may be at least partially determined by the genetic program of the individual (2).

Even though the digital operation may go on without word pairing and have its origin in the genetic substrate of the central nervous system, unless this operation is paired with words, it loses efficiency in communication and in recall. If the digital operation is not coupled with socially conditioned signs and symbols, it is difficult to cue recall.

O. Mandelstam is credited with a quotation that beautifully illustrates this need for word cueing. "I have forgotten the word I intended to say, and my thought, unembodied, returns to the realm of shadows [(11), p. 180]."

Evolution of Language   Until about 150,000 years ago all interorganismic communication was probably on a presymbolic basis. Between 150,000 and 50,000 years ago, the central nervous system of humans reached sufficient capacity to negotiate in abstractions (7). This meant a moving away from sign language to symbolic communication, the use of signs as symbols. It was at that time that human communication became quantitatively and perhaps qualitatively differentiated from all other animal species. We had begun to toy with the tool that would have enormous impact on our subsequent existence. This tool was the abstract word. Although we may be continuing our anatomical evolution, our social evolution, which began at that time, is progressing on a much more rapid scale. The words we began to use were also undergoing an evolutionary process.

Laird has compared a word with an amoeba.

An amoeba is a formless thing which takes many shapes. It moves by thrusting out an arm and flowing into the arm. It multiplies by pulling itself into two without permanently diminishing the original. So with words. A meaning may develop on the periphery of the body of meanings associated with the word and shortly this tentacle has grown to such proportion that it dwarfs all other meanings [8, p. 68].

Loren Eiseley describes the evolution of language rather poetically.

It was a struggle for symbolic communication, for in this new social world communication meant life. The world of instinct was passing. The emergent creature was not whole, was not made truly human until in infancy the dreams of the group, the social constellation amidst which his own orbit was cast had been implanted into the waiting receptive substance of his brain. . . . He was becoming something the world had never seen before. A dream animal, living at least partially within a secret universe of his own creation and sharing that secret universe in his head with other similar heads. Symbolic communication had begun. Man had escaped out of the eternal present of the animal world into the knowledge of past and future [5, pp. 120–121].

Pavlov was one of the first to conceptualize language as a learned or conditioned phenomenon. He believed that the abstract or symbolic communication process followed the same rules as sign language. He did, nevertheless, differentiate the two phenomena into the first signal system and the second signal system. He described the second signal system or symbolic communication as a

special socially conditioned addition which shows a qualitative peculiarity. The addition is connected with labor and social activity, concerns the speech function, and introduces a new principle into the activity of the cerebral hemispheres constituting the second signal of reality typical only of man. By daily combining the various stimuli of the first signal system under conditions of coordination with the environment a word becomes a real and significant conditioned stimulus and constitutes the basis of a complex system of interhuman signals. . . . In addition verbal stimuli act as an abstraction from reality and admit generalizations thus forming the specifically human higher thinking. Abstractions from reality characteristic of the second signal system are achieved because the image of objects and actions expressed in words and ideas replaces their concrete effect on the organism [14, pp. 15–16].

Even though symbolic language is at least in part a learned phenomenon, the human animal appears to have a genetic predisposition to this type of biologic functioning with an enormous drive to acquire these communication skills.

Symbolic Speech and the Ability to Predict

As a child develops the ability to verbalize abstractions through the use of symbolic speech, the child is not only able to codify perceptive inputs that can be compared with memories of previous perceptions, but is better able to make predictions about future perceptive inputs. This ability to generalize and to plan for future contingencies is most highly developed in the human animal. The foregoing process not only increases a child's knowledge of the environment but provides a sense of continuity between previous events and anticipated future events. Simultaneously with increasing knowledge, the child develops abstractions about himself and the relation of his self-system to the environment.

Piaget implies that the child

must develop the symbolic function of representation which is necessary for both progressive subject–object differentiation and cognition that transcends the spatio-temporal bonds of immediate experience of acts and events. Finally, the child must use representation as a means of conventional social communication so that his thinking becomes integrated with the ways of life and thinking of his community. . . . In summary the theory maintains that the emergent genetic function that determines and gives significance to human development is the intention to know. This intentionality is reflected by the child's progressive tendency to construct rather than to mirror or react to a pre-formed reality as he develops. The emergent activity subserving this end is representation, or symbolic operations [9, pp. 131, 112].

The Use of Words—A Group Phenomenon

Self-conceptualization, which reaches its pinnacle in the human animal, gives us a unique and enormous advantage over other forms of life; however, our dependency on digitalized symbolic operations has some liabilities. One of the liabilities of our growing dependence on symbolic operations or our use of the second signal system is the distortion that occurs when perceptive inputs or thought processes are forced into the digital paradigm of words. This is particularly relevant to those persons involved in research and clinical activities. Once we have developed a cognitive set, that is, a linear arrangement of our digital operation, we avoid dissonance by making perceptive inputs fit the stereotyped patterns we were predicting. This is especially evident in the study of human behavior, where various abstractions or diagnostic labels influence to some degree the way we perceive the behavioral patterns we are studying.

For example, a mental health professional observes a person exhibiting a certain pattern of behavior and labels the individual a schizophrenic. This stereotyping may focus attention on some behavioral patterns and exclude others. Schizophrenia, as a label, is a distortion implying a defined entity even though each person exhibiting schizophrenic behavior is different from any other person exhibiting schizophrenic behavior.

Other examples of social significance can be seen in the following stereotypic statements: *He is a Negro. She's only a housewife. Act like a man. She's just a kid.*

Perhaps the most ominous products of our symbolic operation are the illusions or delusions that develop in the process of self-conceptualization. By the use of symbols and abstractions we conceptualize ourselves as unique individuals, and by our digital operation we further qualify ourselves as good, bad, intelligent, attractive, independent, or whatever. The data concerning ouselves, acquired via social interactions is continually used as a reference point in processing subsequent data.

In differentiating ourselves by the use of this symbolic operation, we are using symbols that require consensual validation. The very use of words is a group phenomenon. A word has meaning only if several people agree to its interpretation. Of course, individuals can develop neologisms that have meaning only to themselves, but the overuse of this type of abstraction would exclude them from many social interchanges and markedly limit their data-sharing activities.

Alienated Dependency of Man

Those individuals who survive in society have been conditioned to use symbols that can be validated. Therefore, we have the paradox of an individual who differentiates himself from the group by a process that is dependent on the group. This paradox we have termed *alienated dependency*.

Whether humans were group animals in the prelanguage stage of our evolution is uncertain. The use of words now forces us to belong to a group. Our behavior is now almost totally dependent on our past and present social communication systems. Just as our physiological development is dependent upon our genetic heritage, much of our behavioral patterns are derived from the social milieu in which we develop and live. One might toy with the analogy of a word as being to our social milieu what a gene is to our physiological program. In either case, the individual has very little choice in his heritage. We are all at the mercy of a vast symbolic operation. This point has been emphasized very well by Marshall McLuhan in his work describing the effect of various communications media on human behavior (12).

Transmission of Information

Words are not time-locked. Our present communications systems are influenced by words recorded by individuals from the remote past. Since the advent of recording systems, we have progressed from pictographs to the written word to audio and visual recordings, which have vastly increased the information flowing into our immediate social system. Words may have originally been used by us as a tool, but one has the uncomfortable feeling that the servant has now become the master and that we are becoming victims of rather depersonalized word systems. Paraphrasing Pinter, "We have created the word and in a certain way the word finds its own life, stares at us, is obdurate, and more often than not defeats us" (13).

Even though we have evolved a rather elaborate second signal system of communication, we carry with us all the other coding phenomena of the animal kingdom. We would like to believe that learning has now superceded innate codes or instincts in man, but the instincts still persist. Reconciling the old codes with the new is not always easy. If we forget that the use of symbols, abstractions, and words is a biologic process, the oversight leads to separating language and symbolic coding operations from other physiologic coding phenomena, that is, the psyche (mind) versus the soma (body) antinomy. Our linguistic systems of coding data are influenced by all other systems in our body.

Occasionally, our conditioned patterns of communication do or do not accurately reflect our emotional state, affective tone, or physiologic internal milieu. This may lead to paradoxical situations, miscommunications, and a lack of predictability in human relationships.

Importance of Both Analog and Digital Data-Processing in Human Communication

To return to our model of analog and digital programming of data, we will assert that human communication is dependent on both these modes. The analog mode of data processing is reflected in the facial expressions, intonations, and other nonverbal activity, whereas the digital operation is expressed in words.

Should an individual impart one set of information with his nonverbals and a differing set of data with his verbals, the paradox results in communication difficulties. In human interaction, the synchronization of these two modes of communication is mandatory for the smooth flow of information among individuals. For example, if a person states he is not angry even though his grimace, tight fists, and clinched teeth give nonverbal messages that he is angry, the receiver of these communications may have difficulty in integrating the contradictory messages.

It would appear that the nonverbal elements of communication which stem from the analogic operation are phylogenetically older than the digitalized symbolic operation. The importance of nonverbal communication has been emphasized by Lorenz (19). Darwin's work on facial expressions (4) and work by Ekman (6) indicate that this mode of communication or expression has more continuity throughout the animal kingdom and cross-cultural reliability than the more recently learned symbolic operation which is a readout of the digital system.

Summary

By coupling the units of our digital operation with words, gestures, and designs, we developed language. By this mode of communication, including signs and symbols, we partially escaped from the rigid limitation of innate genetic codes and stimulus locked experiential learning. We became more aware of our individuality through information shared with others. The symbolic operation allowed information to be transmitted between individuals remote from each other in time and space. The information programmed within the individual from internal and external sources is arranged by his digital operation in a sequential order that differentiates the individual from his environment. The use of language augments this differentiation, resulting in the development of a self system, which is used as a reference point in coding subsequent data. The self-referencing system permits us to conceptualize our information systems as unique with delineated boundaries.

References

1. Brown, R., *Words and things:* An introduction to language. New York: Macmillan, 1958, p. 193.

2. Chomsky, N. *Language and mind.* New York: Harcourt Brace Jovanovich, 1972.

3. Chomsky, N. Linguistic contributions to the study of mind: Future. In P. Adams (Ed.), *Language in thinking.* Hammondsport, England: Penguin Books, 1972. Pp. 323–363.

4. Darwin, C. The expression of the emotions. In T. Parsons, E. Shils, K. Naegele, and J. Pitts (Eds.), *Theories of society: Foundations of modern sociological theory,* Vol. II. New York: Free Press, 1961. Pp. 1168–1169.

5. Eiseley, L. *The immense journey.* New York: Vintage Books, 1959.

6. Ekman, P. Face muscles talk every language. *Psychology Today,* 1975, 9(4), 35–39.

7. Hockett, C. *Man's place in nature.* New York: McGraw-Hill, 1973. P. 412.

8. Laird, C. *The miracle of languages.* Greenwich, Connecticut: Fawcett Publications, 1953.

9. Langer, J. *Theories of development.* New York: Holt, Rinehart and Winston, 1969.

10. Lorenz, K. *On aggression.* New York: Harcourt, Brace, Jovanovich, 1963.

11. Mandelstam, O. In T. Vygotsky, Thought and word, In P. Adams (Ed.), *Language in thinking,* Hammondsport, England: Penguin Books, 1972. Pp. 180–213.

12. McLuhan, M. *Understanding media.* New York: McGraw-Hill, 1964.

13. Pinter, H. Some remarks made by the playwright in accepting the Shakespeare Prize of the University of Hamburg on June 4, 1970.

14. Platonov, K., *The word as a physiological and therapeutic factor.* Moscow: Foreign Language Publishing House, 1959.

15. Van Lawick, J. The behavior of chimpanzees in their natural habitat, *American Journal of Psychiatry*, 1973, *130*, 1–12.

16. Vygotsky, L. Thought and word. In P. Adams (Ed.), *Language in thinking.* Hammondsport, England: Penguin Books, 1972. Pp. 180–213.

17. Wilson, E. Animal communication, *Scientific American*, 1972, *227*(3), 53–60.

**Suggested
Readings**

Aaronson, D., and Rieber, R. (Eds.). *Developmental psy-cholinguistics and communication disorders.* New York: New York Academy of Sciences, 1975.

Adams, P. (Ed.). *Language in thinking.* Hammondsport, England: Penguin Books, 1972.

Alloway, T., Krames, L., and Pliner, P. *Communication and affect: A comparative approach.* New York: Academic Press, 1972.

Brown, R. *Words and things: An introduction to language.* New York: Macmillan, 1958.

Cassirer, E. Language in the phase of sensuous expression. In T. Parsons, E. Shils, K. Naegele, and J. Pitts (Eds.), *Theories of society: Foundations of modern sociological theory,* Vol. II. New York: Free Press, 1961. Pp. 1170–1178.

Gould, J. Honey bee recruitment: The dance-language controversy, *Science,* 1975, *189*(4204), 685–693.

Mead, G. From gesture to symbol. In T. Parsons, E. Shils, K. Naegele, and J. Pitts (Eds.), *Theories of society: Foundations of modern sociological theory,* Vol. II. New York: Free Press, 1961. Pp. 999–1004.

Miller, P. *Sense and symbol: A textbook of human behavioral science.* New York: Harper & Row, 1967.

Oldfield, R., and Marshall, J. (Eds.), *Language.* Hammondsport, England: Penguin Books, 1973.

Piaget, J. Language and thought from the genetic point of view. In P. Adams (Ed.), *Language in thinking.* Hammondsport, England: Penguin Books, 1972. Pp. 170–179.

Piaget, J. On intellectual growth. In T. Parsons, E. Shils, K. Naegele, and J. Pitts (Eds.), *Theories of society: Foundations of modern sociological theory,* Vol. II. New York: Free Press, 1961. Pp. 830–834.

Piaget, J. *The origins of intelligence in children.* New York: W. W. Norton, 1952.

Reichenbach, H. *Elements of symbolic logic.* New York: Free Press, 1947.

Shannon, C. A mathematical theory of communication. In R. Oldfield and J. Marshall (Eds.), *Language.* Hammondsport, England: Penguin Books, 1968. Pp. 257–262.

White, L. The symbol: The origin and basis of human behavior. In J. Jennings and E. Hoebel (Eds.), *Readings in anthropology,* 3rd ed. New York: McGraw-Hill, 1972. Pp. 315–321.

**Suggested
Questions**

1. Explain the difference between signs and symbols in human communication.

2. What does Chomsky postulate about the difference between the language of the human animal and that of other animals?

3. Explain one effect of not coupling the digital operation with words.

4. Explain Pavlov's use of the phrase "second signal system."

5. State two functions that children can accomplish as they develop their ability to verbalize abstractions.

6. Give an example of how our symbolic operations may influence the way we perceive an individual.

7. What is the meaning of the sentence, "The very use of words is a group phenomenon?"

8. Explain the phrase "alienated dependency" with reference to man.

9. What may happen if we forget that the use of symbols, abstractions, and words is a biological phenomenon?

10. How is human communication dependent on both the analogic and digital programming of data?

11. What does the self-referencing system permit us to do?

5 Evolution of the Self System

The question, "How does it feel to be you" is forever unanswerable by any method of science, not for lack of instrumentation, but in principle, because if you were told that my inner consciousness was somehow projected on yours, you could never verify the truth of this statement.

Anatol Rapoport, 1976 p. 231

Self-Differentiation through the Evolutionary Process

In the previous chapters we discussed biologic evolution and systems theory. We divided the data-processing systems of the human organism into a bimodal framework—the analog and digital coding systems. We used the term *mind* when referring to brain research and the attempts to localize this phenomenon.

At this point in our study, we might state that we all see ourselves as having a brain, a mind, being conscious, and having the ability to think (process data). We also see ourselves as being different and unique. We develop a *self system*.

From the moment of conception, each person is different from any other, owing to endogenous information (genetic codes). This difference is augmented by data an individual acquires from the environment. Information codes from genetic and experiential sources influence the individual's self-concept. This concept includes physical appearance (blonde, brown-eyed, thin, tall), cognitive skills (bright, slow, average, genius), social acceptability (friendly, shy, leader, recluse), and other attributes. The individual becomes "conscious" of himself.

Consciousness is a rather nebulous word used to denote a coordinated system of information processing and organization. Levels of consciousness vary, depending on the sophistication or complexity of the information-processing system. In all animals consciousness is dependent upon the state of arousal of the central nervous system.

In studying human behavior, we frequently use the term *conscious* to denote that data that are organized or coordinated with data contained in the concept we have of ourselves. With this format we say, "I am conscious" or "not conscious" of certain events, depending on whether information relates to the self system and not on whether perceptive information enters an alert central nervous system.

For example, we are only occasionally conscious of the pressure of our clothing on our bodies even though perceptive data from our sense organs concerning this pressure is continually delivering information to our central nervous system. We say we are not conscious of certain stimuli but, at the same time, we are not unconscious, that is, comatose.

We must be careful, when we use the word *conscious*, to indicate which way we are using it

1. In a general sense, to denote the individual's total state of alertness.
2. In a specific sense, to indicate that an individual is aware of certain events.

Our consciousness in both the general and specific sense depends on the state of arousal of our central nervous systems. The quantity and quality of information processed in an optimal state of consciousness is also dependent on genetically determined potentials and experiential factors.

To illustrate, a person with genetically induced defects in his information-processing system (for example, Down's syndrome, or mongolism) will have diminished ability to program data (learn). Similarly, an individual with no genetic defects will have difficulty in learning if his environment is impoverished (for example, a person who has never seen a cash register will have difficulty understanding it on his first encounter).

We can state, therefore, that our *self-consciousness* (all the information relating to ourselves), is the product of biologic and social evolution. To be our present "selves," we must have

1. Our evolved central nervous systems.
2. The stimulus-related experiences we have acquired from our particular evolved cultures.

Most of us are quite willing to accept the theory of evolution when it pertains to our various organ systems, including our central nervous system, but when we attempt to conceptualize our "selves" as evolving abstractions of data-processing systems, we become insecure. We find it difficult to appreciate the self system as a dynamic and constantly evolving conceptual phenomenon.

Evolution does not itself create anything (7). Evolution is the process by which material already present is rearranged in different organizational patterns. It would seem, then, that the mind, which "contains" the concept of self, evolves from relationships among the cellular activities (chemical and electrical) of the brain.

Sherrington says that, "the connection of the brain with mind seems to rest on the organization of the brain, and that organization is cell-organization. An observer's only means of inferring mind, other than his own which he experiences not, is behaviour . . . [7, pp. 208–209]."

The human is a product of biologic and social reproduction. As George Gaylord Simpson explains it,

Man is one of the millions of results of this material process. He is another species of animal, but not just another animal. He is unique in peculiar and extraordinarily significant ways. He is probably the most self-conscious of organisms, and quite surely the only one that is aware of his own origins, of his own biological nature. He has developed symbolization to a unique degree and is the only organism with true language. This makes him also the only animal who can store knowledge beyond individual capacity and pass it on beyond individual memory [8, p. 13].

Since biologic evolution has, in some degree, biased the manner in which perceptions are coded, there seems to be a continuity, or predictable relationship, of the data coding system among various cultures and between the present culture and previous cultures. This similarity gives the illusion that data from previous cultures is inborn in an individual's memory banks. Perhaps this genetically structured potential in the human for analog to digital conversion of data is very similar to what Jung speculatively called the *collective unconscious* (4).

Self, Ego, Identity, and Personality

The complex interacting open system of data we term the self system has been abstractly termed in other contexts as *self, ego, identity,* or *personality.* Although various authors differ in their description of this phenomenon, there is a tendency to concretize or make a closed system of this dynamic activity, that is, to conceptualize it as an identity like the brain, liver, or heart. The use of this concrete approach colors our speculations about the evolution of the human self.

When did the animal that we now call human begin to evolve the self system? Or did this phenomenon occur spontaneously when the central nervous system reached sufficient capacity to allow abstract thinking? When did our digital operation and language allow us the ability to conceptualize our "selves" as unique and different from our environment? When the first humans accomplished self-realization, were they as rigid in defining the boundaries of their self systems as we are today? If so, we may describe our discovery of the "self" as analogous to our discovery of the use of stone tools.

This concrete way of conceptualizing the self can be demonstrated by the following tongue-in-cheek short story.

The Self

Once upon a time, a primate stumbled upon a self which he kept for his own and shared with his mate. He continued to polish the self until it became his chief preoccupation. At first he kept it in his cave but when he could contain his pride no longer, he and his wife and their children, who were also now attached to the self, began to carry it about when they visited with other primates.

At first the other primates didn't notice how self-centered the little family was but their dedication to self made them more and more self-serving until the other primates began to complain that they were becoming self-conscious, a very uncomfortable feeling. They tried to persuade the family to become less selfish and rejoin the group as before.

The family declared that they considered their self to be the most precious possession in the world so they decided to take their self and leave the group. Unfortunately, they had taken such good care of their self that it had grown so large it was difficult for a single family member to carry it.

They began to argue as to who would carry the self which they all agreed belonged to the entire family. When it looked as if the family were about to fight over who had the right to carry the self or who was least able to carry it, the father, after much deliberation, decided to divide the self into six parts, one each for himself, his wife, and their four children. This allowed everyone to have a self, and, at night, around the fire they could put the parts of the self back together and have a family self which they all agreed would be a beautiful act of sharing their selves.

As the family wandered, some parts of the self continued to grow, probably due to the greater care of the individuals who carried it, while other parts stayed the same size or shrunk a little. This began to cause a problem when the family gathered for a self-merger. The parts no longer fit.

This asymmetry of parts led to quarrels as to who was causing the family self to become misshapen. Those whose selves had grown boasted that they were contributing more than those whose selves had not grown. Those with a smaller self complained that it was selfish of the others to boast when it was their self-indulgence that caused the family self to be unstable.

The mother began to realize that this self-deception was disrupting her family and threatened self-annihilation. Her threat caused the family to quiet down temporarily but their self-interest grew more rapidly in silence than when they were sharing their selves with one another. Finally, some of the children began not to present their selves at the family gatherings, and, as they began to share their selves with more of their peers outside the family, they began to mate with others who were interested in their selves.

A strange phenomenon began to appear when a family was established. The selves, and there were many now, grew rapidly for awhile but then the selves were fragmented to keep peace and each family member took his self out of the total family self.

After several generations, all the families in the area became self-oriented. Self became the major constellation in marriage, family, and community esteem. The primate with the largest self would become the leader and those with smaller selves would dedicate their selves to the leader, at least for as long as his self appeared to be growing.

Whenever the leader's self-esteem grew beyond the size of his actual self, trouble began, especially when leaders of other groups developed their own self-pride. This pride often grew to self-righteousness so that each group felt their self to be superior to all others.

Other groups who realized their weakness stayed out of conflict by self-sacrifice and self-denial. Still others, seeing the dilemma, sat miserably by, involved in self-recrimination.

The process continued despite all the difficulties. Everyone admired the self-made man. Self-realization became part of civilization.

Occasionally, prophets would pass through their villages decrying selfishness, advising self-control, or actually advocating that there was something more important than self, that self-interest was a detriment to gaining this important something. In the majority of primates, this kind of talk made them insecure about their selves and again reaffirming their self-confidence and self-assurance, they attacked the prophets and occasionally killed one.

There were a few who became so caught up in the prophet's teaching that they tended to lose their selves or neglect self-concern and they contended that they were happier. Some actually appeared that way. Others seemed to be more involved in self-deception and rigid self-denial while simultaneously becoming more self-righteous.

For the majority, the selves became more important until all activity was selfish. Their selves were elevated to the roles of ruthless tyrants and self-conceit caused continual frustration and misery.

The people became so miserable that groups began to blame other groups more than ever before and finally, as self-interest groups congealed into larger and larger groups, there were at least two huge opposing groups. Both groups blamed the self of the other group and, after much preparation, set out in a major war of self-destruction.

When the war was over, many of the primates were dead and their selves shattered. Those who remained gathered up the fragments of their selves and swore this time to exercise more self-control.

Slowly, slowly, the process began again—and again. At some time during the ages, persons learned to counterfeit selves so that there was often confusion. Even today many persons spend time and money in search of their true or real selves.

It seems much more productive from our point of view to conceive of the self system as the property of related data, analogous to the crystalline properties resulting from atomic relationships in a grain of salt. The self system then expands if data fit into a pattern with the previous data organization.

Comparison of Theories

As we continue to attempt, through research and clinical activities, to define the processes that result in the development of self-awareness, we are becoming more convinced that the self system (personality, ego, identity) is a working construct, an "as if" paradigm rather than a concrete entity. Several theories and opinions have been advanced concerning the self.

John Eccles believes that the conscious self is in liaison with if not constructed by the "specific linguistic and ideational zones of the dominant hemisphere [1, p. 214]."

Freud was one of the first to interpret the data-processing systems of the human brain on a bimodal basis. He conceptualized basic instinctual drives under an umbrella that he termed the *id*. This is very similar to the analogic data programming system. The part of the digital programming system associated with the self system he termed the *ego* (3).

The ego psychologists and developmental psychologists have placed heavy emphasis on how we differentiate ourselves. Erik Erikson delineated eight stages that the human needs to negotiate in developing and maintaining a stable self system or *identity* (2).

The Freudians and neo-Freudians focused on how unconscious material could be made conscious, that is, how analogic data are digitalized and cross-referenced with the self system.

Piaget has documented the development of self-differentiation in his study of children as they develop what he terms *formal operations,* in which the conceptualization of their external milieu progresses beyond stimulus-bound phenomena. For example, the child begins to appreciate that similar quantities of water may look different depending on the shapes of their containers. In children, the use of a linguistic code occurs about the same time that a child differentiates self from environment (5).

It would seem that the use of linguistic codes facilitates, if not causes, the development of a self system. The use of the first-person pronoun and the coupling of possessive pronouns and self-qualifying adjectives allowing the compilation of digitalized data referring to the perceivers indicate the evolution of a self-system.

The Search for Information to Reify the Self

Once the individual begins to view himself as being separate from others and as being unique, he then begins a continual search for information that will validate his self-concept. Man's aptitude for coding data is complemented by his drive to obtain information or to process new data, a facility Piaget termed the *intentionality to know.* By way of metaphor, we might say that the human brain exhibits an appetite for information, or data hunger, analogous to the animal's drive for food.

Animals exert energy in order to obtain food (energy). The larger the physiologic apparatus, the more energy necessary to keep it functioning. An example of this is seen in the unfortunate obese person whose enlarged body tissues increase the need for food in an increasing upward spiral.

The human brain, with its hypertrophied capacity for analog and digital coding of data, drives the individual to seek more data. The more data programmed, the greater the individual's ability to incorporate new information.

For example, students do not start out with all the knowledge related to their fields of study. They go through an educational process which feeds increasingly more complex data into their memory banks. The more information they program, the greater is their ability to code new data and to store it for retrieval.

The most unbiased form of data hunger is seen in the curiosity of children. As information moves from children's experience through their analog coding apparatus into the digital operation, they learn to pair the latter with the words of their cultural system. Perceptive inputs and data processing depend on differentiation. This predicates a subject–object dichotomy so that children soon begin to program the difference between the perceiver and the perceived.

We may say, then, that the self system is a fluid and continually changing relationship of coded data used as a reference point to differentiate the perceiver from the perceived. Although this process may originate from our drive to understand, or our information hunger, it is accelerated and biased as the data processed further differentiate us from our environment.

By extrapolation, and through a process of linear logic, the individual begins to conceptualize his self system as not only unique but finite. He becomes aware that he has a beginning and an end and that certain situations may terminate his existence. Since individual and species survival seem to be properties of all living systems, the drive to survive is now paired with the drive to know. This not only quickens the pace of information gathering, it also narrows the field so that the individual selectively searches for information that has bearing on his survival and the enhancement of his existence.

The person who is trained to use language as a source of data sharing among other persons now frantically exchanges data at every opportunity with those in his environment. The compulsion for exchanging information makes man one of the most group-dependent species in the animal world. Lewis Thomas has stated,

> The human brain is the most public organ on the face of the earth, open to everything, sending out messages to everything. To be sure, it is hidden away in bone and conducts internal affairs in secrecy, but virtually all the business is the direct result of thinking that has already occurred in other minds. We pass thought around, from mind to mind, so compulsively and with such speed that the brains of mankind often appear, functionally, to be undergoing fusion. This is, when you think about it, really amazing. The whole dear notion of one's own Self—marvelous old free-willed, free-enterprising, autonomous, independent, isolated island of Self—is a myth [9, p. 142].

Individual Data Selection

The self system, which is continuous, but changing throughout a lifetime, is constantly influenced by new data, but it, in turn, influences how the data will be perceived and programmed. Certain bits of data that do not fit the circumscribed self system will be excluded or, as Freud might have termed, *repressed,* whereas other data that fit and modify the self system in a way that increases the individual's security are readily acceptable and are easily synchronized with data already in the self system (*ego syntonic* in Freudian terminology).

The "as if" proposition termed self is used as a reference point in processing information in an empirically predictable sequence. In addressing the self system of an individual, we may again use the analogy of a crystal. Various roles and patterns of behavior are related to each other in a changing but predictable manner. Predictable relationships give the individual the illusion of stability and autonomy. We are able to predict how we will respond to a given bit of data. If the prediction is not accurate and the response does not fit our self system, we may excuse the variance by stating, "I was just not myself." As individuals, we spend a great deal of time trying to understand what our "real selves" are or why other people do not appreciate us for ourselves.

These prized self systems are not only influenced by the behavior of others, present and past, but by the individual's own behavior, which biases his future behavior.

The emotions, or affective tones, of the individual may be considered to be a readout of a feedback relationship among the analog and digital coding systems and those systems concerned with arousal and emotion (for example, the reticular activating system and the limbic system). Emotions color cognitive functions, and vice versa. The fluctuating relationships between the analog and digital system, that is, the A–D ratio, influence the conglomeration of data we term a self.

There seems little doubt that reproductive and vegetative systems are continually interacting with the data programming activity of the central nervous system and probably have a marked influence on the patterns of behavior incorporation in our self systems. Freudian theory often emphasizes libidinal (sexual) energy as the major driving force. A more flexible approach would be to consider all of these systems interacting with the activating and emotional systems and the self system, resulting in a behavioral readout that is a composite of these interactions.

As each person further delineates his own boundaries, he adopts standardized relationships with social institutions to help him in this endeavor. These relationships are evident when the individual liaisons himself with social institutions concerned with status, wealth, religion, education, occupation, etc. Each bit of information selected by the individual during these activities makes him seem unique and allows others to identify him.

For instance, a case history used in a clinical situation may begin, "This is a 43-year-old white Protestant married male, father of three children, who is currently employed as president of a local bank." We now know the sex, age, religion, marital and family status, race, and occupation of the patient. We may also infer that the individual is fairly well educated, literate, and an influential member of the community. This man's self system is being reified and delineated not only by himself but by those who have acquired the selected information about his self system. He has a partially defined identity.

By using these socially validated or stereotypical descriptive phrases, the individual is, to some extent, differentiated from others. This reification may seem clinically efficient. However, the data given imply that his self system is closed. There is no indication of the presence or absence of flexibility in the system to incorporate continuous data input, which is of enormous clinical significance.

Since we define the individual as a pattern of interacting coded information, the term self may be applied to the interaction of coded information exchanged in a group of individuals whether the group be a family, community, or cultural system.

Like the individual self, the family self has many properties of a myth as defined by *Webster's*. The history of a family can be described as "a usually traditional story of ostensibly historical events that serves to unfold part of the world view of a people or explain a practice, belief, or natural phenomenon [10, p. 762]."

Consequences of Differentiation

Most of us are rather proud of our individual and family selves and think that we are unique types of creation. We are possessive about the phenomena we call our "selves," and, if these are in any way questioned, we reply, "That's just me," implying that this statement is adequate to explain all our activities of which we are not ashamed.

It would appear, then, that the establishment and maintenance of a self system carries with it two necessities: (a) to defend that system, and (b) to augment it by appropriately selected data. The individual spends a lifetime expanding and reifying that entity known as the self, and also becomes aware of situations which may terminate existence and of the transiency and tenuousness of his delineated self system. So the individual strives for security by data sharing.

The shared digital and analog operation of a family is similar to the self system of an individual. When the data emitted from the analog and digital systems of each family member is synchronized so that rapid predictable data processing occurs, the self system of the individual is, to some extent, merged into what might be termed a *family self system*. This provides a buffer and a type of security for the individual self system.

Conclusion

The self is a working construct, a fluid base of reference we use in programming information. It must be constantly tuned to function in harmony with the information processed in all systems. When the data from an individual's environment do not validate the patterns of behavior composing his self system, the individual may become anxious and exhibit various fight–flight patterns. All animals, when threatened, may attempt to survive via innate or learned fight–flight patterns of behavior.

The human animal has, in addition to a need for survival, the need to protect the focus of his information coding system, that is, his self system. Two factors, (a) his information hunger and (b) his need to protect his self system have led to varieties of social institutions including religion, science, law, and art. Through each of these endeavors, we attempt further to differentiate and delineate ourselves and simultaneously avoid self-disillusionment.

In the next chapter, we will focus our attention on our efforts to maintain behavioral homeostasis (equilibrium) through interacting open systems of relationships.

References

1. Eccles, J. *The understanding of the brain.* New York: McGraw-Hill, 1973.

2. Erikson, E. *Childhood and society.* New York: W. W. Norton, 1963.

3. Freud, S. The ego and the superego. In T. Parsons, E. Shils, K. Naegele and J. Pitts (Eds.), *Theories of society: Foundations of modern sociological theory,* Vol. II. New York: Free Press, 1961.

4. Jung, C. *The basic writings of C. G. Jung,* V. DeLaszlo (Ed.) New York: Random House, 1959.

5. Piaget, J. *The origins of intelligence in children.* New York: W. W. Norton, 1963.

6. Rapoport, A. General systems theory: A bridge between two cultures. Third Annual Ludwig von Bertalanffy Lecture. *Behavioral Science,* 1976, *21,* 228–239, p. 231.

7. Sherrington, Sir C. *Man on his nature.* London: Cambridge University Press, 1940.

8. Simpson, G. The world into which Darwin led us. In J. Jennings and E. Hoebel (Eds.), *Readings in anthropology.* New York: McGraw-Hill, 1972.

9. Thomas, L. *The lives of a cell.* New York: Viking Press, 1974.

10. Webster's *New twentieth century dictionary of the English language,* Unabridged. Meriden, Connecticut: William Collins and World, 1975,

Suggested Questions

1. How does each individual see himself?

2. Upon what is consciousness dependent in all animals?

3. Explain two ways of using the term "conscious."

4. What two things must we possess in order to be our present "selves?"

5. Explain the statement, "Evolution does not itself create anything."

6. What gives us the illusion that data from previous cultures is inborn in the individual's memory banks?

7. How does the use of linguistic codes affect the development of a self system?

8. Explain Piaget's phrase "the intentionality to know."

9. Define the term "self system."

10. What makes man one of the most group-dependent species in the world?

11. What factor might cause the self system to exclude certain bits of data?

12. What do predictable relationships give the individual?

13. What are some of the institutions the individual uses to reify his self system, to delineate his own boundaries?

14. List two "necessities" that accompany the establishment and maintenance of a self system.

15. What two factors have led to the establishment of varieties of social institutions?

6 Interpersonal Relationships and Behavioral Homeostasis

There is no sense of "I," as in pride or shame, without its correlative sense of you, or he, or they. Even the miser gloating over his hidden gold can feel the "mine" only as he is aware of the world of men over whom he has secret power; and the case is very similar with all kinds of hid treasure.

Charles H. Cooley, 1922 (3)

Development and Maintenance of a Self

The brain is continually involved in secretory activity—producing transmitters, enzymes and other hormonal substances. The interaction or equilibrium of those chemical substances is the cauldron from which the behavioral readout emanates. We may say that the brain, in conjunction with all other organ systems in the body, secretes behavior. This is analagous to the secretory activity of the kidney the enzyme activity of which, in conjunction with various chemical agents in the perfusing blood flow, results in the output of urine. The secretion (or perhaps excretion) of the brain depends on *informational input* as well as *chemical activity*.

The complex chemical activity of the central nervous system, in dynamic equilibrium with other organ systems, continually screens selected data bits from internal and external sources, resulting in the evolving abstraction we have termed the self system. This screening activity is biased by, and contributes to, the social matrix surrounding the individual.

One form of the social matrix, which provides an excellent vehicle for the birth of the self system, is the family unit. By way of analogy, we might compare the birth of the self system to parturition. In both circumstances, there is a separation of the infant from its mother.

It is doubtful that the immature central nervous system of the child programs much information about the fairly rapid passage from the uterus to the outside world. Even though there is evidence that the process does produce a shock to the infant's physiologic machinery the infant has not developed the digital skills necessary for coding memories and referencing them with a self system. Without linguistic cues for recall, any analogically coded information occurring at this time is beyond present techniques of investigation and must remain a matter of speculation.

In contrast, the birth of the self system and the differentiation of this self from the mother's self occurs over a period of several years, and is usually accomplished by the digital operation and the acquisition of linguistic skills. The differentiation of the self is dependent upon the acquisition of digitally coded memory patterns and various socially validatable roles.

Forcing a child to conform by threatening a loss of security and creating anxiety and guilt could produce a trauma similar to the birth trauma described by Rank (13). Memories and learned patterns acquired during the birth process may be pleasant or unpleasant. These primal memories may influence to some degree subsequent learning patterns and attitudinal sets that will bias the self system and all subsequent information coding. The large variation in the information coded in different self systems makes the information exchange among several self systems extremely complex.

There is a tendency for the study of human behavior to oversimplify the information-exchange system. This may be an attempt to break down the mystique that has surrounded human behavior and to avoid the anthropocentric focus on the human as the center of the universe. This trend was most apparent in some of the early behavioral modification endeavors.

There appears to be some validity in comparing human behavior with the behavior of other animals and in realizing that our information-processing equipment is on a continuum with all living and perhaps nonliving systems. However, we must also appreciate that the evolution of the second signal system, or abstract language, made an enormous quantitative and perhaps qualitative difference between our data-sharing activities and that of other animals.

The thousands of words available for digital coding allow an almost infinite number of combinations. The various combinations of language units are complicated by the emotional or analogic coloring of the language evident in nonverbal gestures and intonations.

Communication, including both analog and digital elements, must be synchronized with memory patterns, the constellation of behaviors in the self system, and the socially validated language system of the individual's culture, all of which are in continual flux and interdependent.

The Group or Social Self

Just as the individual self system evolves, group selves evolve. These include family, community, or cultural systems. The social, or group, self may be considered just as much of an entity for practical purposes as the individual self. One could not be conscious of self without the thought of being differentiated from a more general composite of other self systems.

Cooley expounded the theory of the reflected, or looking-glass, self; the hypothesis that self is imagined only as one's idea of it seems to appear to significant others in his social system:

> *Each to each a looking-glass*
> *Reflects the other that doth pass (3)*

We imagine how we must appear to others and our self-concepts and subsequent behaviors are affected as our perceptions of others fluctuate.

If we consider the general or social self to be in continuous interaction with the individual self system, it is necessary that one be militantly active in order to hold on to the "I" or "me" (the identity, personality, or ego). Therefore, the individual self system is maintained by interaction with other self systems in a reciprocal paradigm designed for validation. These interactions occur within groups that provide the environment for social validation.

Self and the Environment

Since the individual self system could not be defined as such without being differentiated from a general or social self, each person shares with every other person the problem of maintaining behavioral and emotional homeostasis, while balancing a series of simultaneous and often conflicting relationships. The most common social system of interacting open relationships with which almost everyone is familiar is probably that of the family.

The data-processing system of a family or group self provides a broader base for programming contingencies than the individual self. Like the individual self, the family or group self may screen out information that does not fit its data base. This may result in a rigid system that may be extremely effective if the data to be processed remain stable. The empirical efficiency obtained by narrowing tolerance in a living system may decrease the ability to adapt.

If the data-processing system of the family is rigidified and inflexible, new data that occur with increase or decrease in the number of family members or a shift in one or more family members' self systems may be processed inaccurately. A system of data processing that excludes flexibility or tolerance factors soon becomes obsolete.

The various self systems, individual, family, and other societal groups, continuously influence each other. The study of human behavior is in large part the evaluation of how relationships are defined among individual self systems and between the individual self system and larger conglomerate self systems. The definition of relationships delineates the quality and quantity of information that will be shared. They range from formal digital relationships to various analog-to-analog and digital-to-analog combinations of less structured nature.

An example of a primitive data exchange would be the information offered by spontaneous facial expressions, when the readout of the one analogic operation is shared by the analog of another (4,5). The digital–analog relationship is seen in hypnosis, when the digital expression of one self system is allowed to affect directly the analog system of another. These patterns are also seen between the individual and group self systems, for example, charismatic politicians are able to utilize words to evoke an emotional response in their audiences.

The systems involved with emotion and states of arousal directly affect the A–D ratio of information coding as we illustrated in Chapter 3. From clinical observations, it seems that a certain level (or pitch) of arousal is necessary for any marked shift in the organization of the data base of the self concept. This has been noted in less complex data alignments, for example, learned patterns. Pavlov noted that his dogs lost their patterns of conditioned response after being subjected to extreme fear when his laboratory was flooded (12).

Behavioral scientists have noted changes in an individuals's orientation with heightened emotion, especially in group situations, as evidenced by religious conversion or political allegiance. "Brainwashing" techniques have capitalized on this aspect of human behavior (12). An example more cogent to health professionals is the grief work that occurs when an individual sustains the loss of a loved object, resulting in reorientation of the relationships in his environment and the data within his self system.

Communication theorists, especially Jackson, Bateson, and Haley, and those scholars interested in family interactions including Bowen, Lidz, Satir, Wynne, Singer, and Ackerman have all made major contributions to our appreciation of the dynamic interchange between the individual self systems and those of the family and society.

Jackson sees family homeostasis as integral to the treatment of any individual seeking help. Therapeutic intervention must take into consideration the homeostatic unit of the family in order to be effective (7).

Bateson writes extensively about the importance of recognizing the dynamics involved in interacting open systems in treatment of alcoholic patients. He states that, "In no system which shows mental characteristics can any part have unilateral control over the whole. In other words, the mental characteristics of the system are immanent, not in some part, but in the system as a whole [1, p. 316]."

Data Processing and Role Theory

As information is acquired through interpersonal interaction, each human being takes on many roles or behavioral patterns—subsystems within the self system. Each role carries with it a set of expectations. Role systems that can be defined as two or more sets of complementary role expectations (for example, mother–child) are considered the smallest type of social system (11).

Individual roles are composed of elaborate patterns of perceptions and behaviors that a person programs throughout his lifetime. They are predictable patterns of behavior that the individual self system portrays during the interpersonal exchange of data.

All roles are composed of stored information coded by the individual with reference to his self system. The larger the number of roles incorporated in the individual's self system, or identity, the more flexible are his interactions with other persons. This is another way of saying that the broader the data base, the more data there are that can be programmed.

Patterns of coded data, or roles, begin to be incorporated into the individual's self system during childhood. It is of note that the individual develops his self system among multiple self systems, which, in turn, include multiple roles. If the roles of the family are stable, the child is quickly able to incorporate various patterns of data so that his roles are synchronized with the others. Conversely, if family roles are shifting quickly, the child may become anxious and confused, since different patterns of behavior are reinforced positively at one time and negatively at others.

Even in the most stable family constellation, roles are continually shifting. These shifts are often catalyzed by internal and external environmental systems. For example, no sooner does the child learn the productive roles for being a child than he reaches puberty. The roles he used as a child are no longer adequate, and he has to progress to those which the social system demands for adolescence. Roles for peer relationships progress into those for early adulthood, which social pressures require for establishing a predictable adult identity. The progression through various roles and behavioral constellations has been abstractly conceptualized by many students of behavior. Perhaps the model of Erik Erikson, previously noted, has received most wide acclaim in the past.

During adulthood the individual continues to elaborate on his roles as a parent and member of the social system. One self system may include the roles of male, parent, soldier, professional, and others. The survival of various patterns of behavior within the individual's self system is contingent on reinforcement. We are involved in an information-exchange system with those individuals about us. Within our family and other social groups, we are continually seeking validation of our behavior in order to maintain a homeostatic relationship between our self systems and those of others.

The importance of interpersonal realtionships in maintaining an individual identity has been emphasized by many behavioral scientists.

Harry Stack Sullivan devoted his psychiatric career to the study of interpersonal relationships. He believed that interpersonal situations, not the individual, should be the focus of attention. He argued that personality develops throughout the lifetime in the interactions of a given biological substrate, the process of maturation, and all involved relationships (10).

Adolph Meyer, often called the father of American psychiatry, became increasingly involved in developing a holistic biological concept of humanity. Although he approached the study of human behavior from the viewpoint of the individual as a biological unit, he recognized the importance of data related to the patient's life history of interactions in order to treat the individual *psychobiologically*. In his analysis of open systems, Meyer focused almost entirely upon the individual and the larger social system (such as the community) rather than on the smaller unit of the family (9).

Trigant Burrow used the term *phylobiology* in studying the interrelational behavior of the human animal. He was concerned with focusing the attention of the scientific community on research into the complexity of human social reactions (2).

Need for Predictability and Control

One of the major themes in most theories for understanding the interpersonal aspects of human behavior is the need for prediction and control of data emanating from those persons who validate our self-conceptualization. In this endeavor to predict and control, the communication commerce is dependent on smooth integration of data from the analog and digital paradigms of the self system.

The more important one's self system is to others, the more one is able to define relationships with others and control the type and amount of information exchanged. If the producer of a certain pattern of behavior is sufficiently important to others in the exchange system, the producer can bias the exchange by the attention he gives patterns exhibited by others, and he is able to gain their attention with minimal effort.

Every individual makes continual attempts in a given social system to control or influence the quality and quantity of information exchanged. That is, everyone feels more secure when he defines or shares in the definition of relationships.

Relationships may be defined in many ways. Haley states,

If one took all the possible kind of communicative behavior which two people might interchange, it could be roughly classified into behavior which defines a relationship as symmetrical and behavior which defines a relationship as complementary. A symmetrical relationship is one where two people exchange the same type of behavior. Each person will initiate action, criticize the other, offer advice, and so on. This type of relationship tends to be competitive; if one person mentions that he has succeeded in some endeavor, the other person points out that he has succeeded in some equally important endeavor. The people in such a relationship emphasize their symmetry with each other.

A complementary relationship is one where the two people are exchanging different types of behaviors. One gives and the other receives, one teaches and the other learns. The two people exchange behaviors which complements, or fits together. One is in a "superior" position and the other in a "secondary" in that one offers criticism and the other accepts it, one offers advice and the other follows it, and so on [6, p. 11].

An example of a symmetrical relationship might be student–student. A complementary relationship might be student–teacher.

The relationship may be defined by physical prowessness, that is, by the size of one individual or the number of individuals desiring control. For example, an adult may intimidate a child or an army may subjugate a village. Dominance and control are often more subtle and more analogous to commerce than to war. Information is exchanged or bartered in a reciprocal producer–consumer arrangement (as in, "I will validate your behavior if you will validate mine.").

In family constellations, where larger self systems help to pattern individual self systems, the codes through which information is exchanged may shift from one mode to the other rapidly. The more predictable these shifts are, the more stable the family self system is.

The two fluctuating modes of data sharing (analog and digital) may be utilized to exchange information that defines the relationship among participants.

In a parent–child interaction, the parent may control the relationship with a child by sending messages in any combination of the bimodal pattern, that is, the parent may use the digital to command and the analog (facial expression and intonations) to communicate pleasure or displeasure. If the two modes of communication do not transmit the same message the receiver is confronted with a paradox. The readout of the analog (nonverbal) communicates one message and the digital (verbal), the opposite. For example, a parent may admonish a child not to study too hard, but smile while delivering the reprimand, indicating admiration of the child's industry.

Because family and social self systems need to predict the behavior of their individual units, pressure is applied to make the individual conform to these predictions. The individual perceives this pressure as expectations. These expectations are often incorporated into the individual self system, that is, what he expects or requires of his own behavior. Claiming to have an inferiority complex may be a way of stating that "I am anxious about fulfilling expectations of myself and others."

A type of anxiety in not meeting expectations is called *embarrassment*. Embarrassment-prone, or shy, individuals may not feel inferior, but the converse, that is, they feel their behavior to be so important to their self systems and that of the group that they are unwilling to exhibit any behavior that they fear might not meet the expectations of themselves and others.

Expectations are important in shaping and regulating human behavior. We may speculate that the expectations of others are major regulating factors in the development and maintenance of self systems.

An example of expectations as a regulating force on behavior can be seen in the dress of school children. The effect of peer pressure with reference to a child's dress patterns has caused frustration in both children and parents. If every peer is wearing white tube socks, the child may exhibit anxiety if he does not conform to this standard. He may feel isolated or different at school if he wears what his parents choose (which may have been the dress of the day when they were children).

Peer pressure or social reinforcement seems often more important in shaping behavior than other types of reward systems. Like other animals, the human may have his behavior conditioned using food or pain (for example, electric shock). However, many children will endure hunger and discomfort to eat food and wear clothes similar to the food and clothing other children are consuming and wearing. A boy will endure extreme cold if it is considered not masculine to wear something over the ears and head. A girl will risk breaking her ankles by wearing high heeled shoes if her peers wear them.

Interpersonal Skills in a Behavioral Economy

The more skillful a person is in acquiring data that validate his ability to perform in any one role, the more likely he is to be comfortable in that role. Individuals are constantly trying to obtain approval for their actions (consensual validation of their behavioral patterns). Those who are assertive in their methods are more likely to be successful in receiving sufficient attention to validate the roles they have selected for themselves.

Group control is more often exerted by those who can recognize the mood or attitude of the group. They perceive a "generalized other" instead of focusing on individual self systems (8). Whatever the goal of the individual, whether to validate his self system with one significant other or with a generalized other (the group), he must participate in an information–exchange system.

This exchange may be conceptualized as a *behavioral economy,* where patterns of behavior are presented and either validated or rejected by other individuals. There is a continual trading of information similar to the exchange of goods in a marketplace.

In the behavioral economy, the medium of exchange is attention. If a person possesses or develops the necessary communication skills and adopts standardized patterns of validation (social mores), he will be able to give and receive sufficient attention to validate most of the roles in his self system at a given time. Standardized patterns of validation within the social system allow the individual to predict the responses of others to his behavior, and promise him the feeling of being accepted and secure if he conforms to these patterns.

To illustrate, around the turn of the century, many people of different cultures immigrated to the United States. They took whatever jobs were available at that time. Many went into the coal mines and steel mills. They worked hard to achieve some kind of security for their children. Hard work was considered a virtue, and to send a child to college was a goal for many of these parents.

Those children of immigrant parents who adopted the standardized patterns of validation within their social systems (that is, went to school, worked hard, made good grades), could predict that the responses of their families would be favorable. The attention given to their behaviors resulted in their feeling accepted and secure.

The success of interpersonal communication techniques in validating the behavioral patterns of our self systems is dependent on the quantity and quality of attention these techniques receive from others. The quantity and quality of attention is a reflection of the emotional state and state of arousal (level or pitch of emotion) of the participants in a behavioral exchange. Since emotion and alertness are analog functions, it is difficult to utilize words that accurately describe them. This results in our using many nebulous abstractions (for example, love, hate, fear, anger) which are difficult to define accurately.

We can arbitrarily divide attention into the following subcategories:

1. Intense concentration.
2. Concern.
3. Amusement.
4. Ridicule.
5. Indifference.

We might have chosen a number of other terms to indicate the strength and valence of emotional arousal in attention. However, our selection would still be arbitrary.

Let us now assign an arbitrary value to each of these categories so that we may rank them on a scale ranging from most acceptable to least acceptable. The cliché, "Best to be loved but better hated than ignored" seems to hold true in our need for attention so we will rank intense concentration as the most acceptable category of attention and indifference as the least acceptable. We will rank concern, amusement, and ridicule between them. Most would agree that concerned attention is more acceptable to their self systems than ridicule, amusement being somewhere in between.

The categories roughly indicate the pitch or level of emotional arousal associated with each level of attention. Using our attention units, we can create a graph that illustrates how attention affects the way relationships are defined in an information exchange in which one person acts (produces) and the other responds (consumes) behavior.

The quality and quantity of attention given in an interpersonal exchange is an indication of the control exercised by the producer or consumer of behaviors. This can be illustrated by Figure 6.1.

If the consumer were indifferent and the producer showing intense concentration we would graph the interaction as being at point F, with the consumer being in control. Conversely, if the producer were indifferent but the consumer intensely involved we would represent their interchanges as being at point G with producer control. These points define an extreme unilateral or complementary relationship.

If both were equally intensely involved we would plot

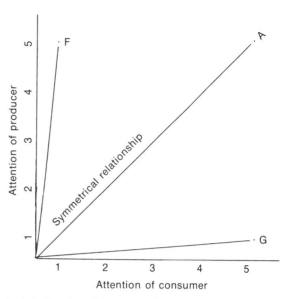

FIGURE 6.1   Attention in an interpersonal exchange as an indicator of control. 5—Intense concentration; 4—Concern; 3—Amusement; 2—Ridicule; 1—Indifference

the relationship at point *A*, where the relationship is equally shared, with neither party having dominant control, that is, a symmetrical relationship. Any point on the graph line labeled "symmetrical relationship" indicates an equal level of emotional arousal in the producer and consumer, whether it be indifference or intense concentration.

Assuming that the producer of a given bit of behavior is successful in obtaining a maximum reaction in the form of passionate or intense attention from his consumer, he will be able to control the exchange as long as he can sustain the attention at that level. However, if his behavioral product begins to attract less energetic attention, he will gradually lose control of the interaction until he finally reaches point *F*, indifference, at which juncture the consumer is fully in control of all exchanges.

Intense concentration, an indicator of consumer or producer involvement, can take the form of hate as well as love. The man and woman who have shared a romance and then find themselves hating each other are just as involved as they were when the intense concentration they are showering on each other took the form of love. Many individuals reach tremendous levels of emotional arousal as they focus on hating some person or some group. If the person who is hated returns the feeling, then the relationship is just as symmetrical as if they exchanged feelings of love and warmth. Having a symmetrical relationship does not imply having a loving relationship. It means that the level of emotional arousal is the same for both persons or groups involved.

The cybernetic quality of the producer–consumer dyad is evident in most interactions, since producers are simultaneously consumers and vice versa. The importance of the level of emotional arousal can also be illustrated by a formula:

$$\frac{\text{Attention obtained}}{\text{Level of emotional arousal}} \times 100 = $$
$$\text{Percentage of efficiency of behavior}$$

The percentage of efficiency is directly proportional to interpersonal skills. A person with limited interpersonal skills has to reach a higher level of emotional arousal to obtain a given amount of attention. Since it takes more effort for him, the emotional pitch will be greater.

For example, the student who has skill and experience in public speaking will not reach nearly the level of emotional arousal when called upon to give an oral presentation as the student who has little practice and questionable skill. The latter may have many more systems of his body involved in an intense interaction. He may have sweaty palms, shortness of breath, and impending diarrhea. In his efforts to gain a maximum favorable reaction from the class in the form of intense concentration, he will have experienced a higher level of emotional arousal with concomitant effects on all his physiological subsystems.

There are, at present, no quantitative units for attention, emotion, or interpersonal skills, and the graph and formula are presented as allegorical illustrations rather than as scientific data arrangements.

Many behavioral patterns can be used to define relationships and control the exchange system. These patterns may include threatened physical violence, the display of a large portfolio of interpersonal skills, the use of symptomatic behavior, and others. The attention received from the consumer of this behavior may be at the quantitative level of intense concentration but it may vary in quality so that we label it fear, hate, love, fascination, or a mixture of these emotions, for example, guilt.

Guilt is an ambivalent combination of emotions, including love, hate, anger, fear, need, and revulsion. This mixture of emotions is appreciated by the analog system but does not allow concise digitalization. The amount of anxiety, anger, need and affection varies in different individuals and in the same individual in different situations, even though the word *guilt* is used as a blanket term, making it widely applicable but rather indefinite.

The individual who transgresses social rules may contend that he feels guilty for the act. A child who displeases his mother may express a similar mixture of feelings under the same word. The insecurity and threatened loss of a source of validation, attention, or affection, may prevent anger from being actively expressed by the individual and others. Since most individuals state that this ambivalent emotion is uncomfortable, some individuals may evoke the feeling in others as a force for modifying their behavior. This evoking of guilt feeling is widespread, in large part due to the social sanctions against more direct aggression.

An individual may plead that he is feeling guilty to modify or ameliorate the responses of others and prevent their behavior from progressing to that of aggression toward him or their withdrawal from exchanging information with him. Pleading guilty is analogous to token submission in aggression-laden interpersonal relationships.

To illustrate, if you agree to meet a friend after one of your classes and you forget to keep the appointment, it might be effective to say, "I feel so awful. I feel so guilty. I don't know how I could have forgotten. I can't imagine what was on my mind. I do feel terribly guilty." Since you already admit to overwhelming feelings of guilt and you submit to your friend, ready for whatever punishment you have implied you deserve, he is less likely to be hostile and is more likely to say, "Well, okay. I was angry at first but you don't have to feel so guilty. Let's just forget it. But don't let it happen again." You have effectively controlled the level of anger and aggression that might have been directed at you had you acted as if the forgotten appointment had had little effect upon you.

Various physiologic symptoms may be utilized to control or bias the information-exchange system and the definition of relationships (for example, "I would live up to your expectations if I were not ill," or "I deserve special attention since I am in pain").

The use of guilt and symptoms in the behavioral

economy of interpersonal relationships has major significance in the study of human behavior and will be addressed in subsequent chapters.

References

1. Bateson, G. *Steps to an ecology of mind.* New York: Ballantine Books, 1972.

2. Burrow, T. *Science and man's behavior: The contribution of phylobiology.* New York: Philosophical Library, 1953.

3. Cooley, C. The social self. In T. Parsons, E. Shils, K, Naegele, and J. Pitts (Eds.), *Theories of society: Foundations of modern sociological theory,* Vol. II. New York: Free Press, 1961. Pp 822–828.

4. Darwin, C. The expression of the emotions. In T. Parsons, E. Shils, K. Naegele, and J. Pitts (Eds.), *Theories of society: Foundations of modern sociological theory,* Vol. II. New York: Free Press, 1961. Pp. 1168–1170.

5. Ekman, P. Face muscles talk every language. *Psychology Today,* 1975, 9(4), 35–39.

6. Haley, J. *Strategies of psychotherapy.* New York: Grune & Stratton, 1963.

7. Jackson, D. The question of family homeostasis. In D. Jackson (Ed.), *Communication, family and marriage.* Palo Alto, California: Science and Behavior Books, 1970. Pp. 1–11.

8. Mead, G. Taking the role of the other. In T. Parsons, E. Shils, K. Naegele, and J. Pitts (Eds.), *Theories of society: Foundations of modern sociological theory,* Vol. I. New York: Free Press, 1961. Pp. 739–740.

9. Mora, G. Adolph Meyer. In A. Freeman, H. Kaplan, and B. Sadock (Eds.), *Comprehensive textbook of psychiatry/II,* Vol. I. Baltimore: Williams and Wilkins, 1975. Pp. 626–632.

10. Mullahy, P. Harry Stack Sullivan. In A. Freedman, H. Kaplan, and B. Sadock (Eds.), *Comprehensive textbook of psychiatry/II,* Vol. I. Baltimore: Williams and Wilkins, 1975. Pp. 598–613.

11. Pitts, J. Introduction. In T. Parsons, E. Shils, K. Naegele, and J. Pitts (Eds.), *Theories of society: Foundations of modern sociological theory.* Vol. II. New York: Free Press, 1961. Pp. 685–716.

12. Sargent, W. *Battle for the mind.* Hammondsport, England: Penguin Books, 1961.

13. Schmitt, A. Otto Rank. In A. Freedman, H. Kaplan, and B. Sadock (Eds.), *Comprehensive textbook of psychiatry/II,* Vol. I. Baltimore: Williams and Wilkins, 1975. Pp. 637–641.

**Suggested
Questions**

1. On what two factors does the "behavioral secretion" of the brain depend?

2. On what two acquisitions does the differentiation of the self depend?

3. What is probably the most common social system of interacting open relationships with which almost everyone is familiar?

4. Explain, briefly, Cooley's theory of the reflected, or looking-glass, self.

5. What is necessary for any marked shift in the organization of the data base of the self concept?

6. What is the smallest type of social system?

7. Of what are roles composed?

8. What might be the effect on a child if family roles are shifting quickly?

9. What are Haley's definitions of symmetrical and complementary relationships? Give an example of each.

10. Give one reason why pressure is applied to make an individual conform to expectations.

11. Discuss the phrase *behavioral economy*.

12. What is the medium of exchange in a behavioral economy?

13. Give your opinion of the attention graph. Do you agree or disagree with the arbitrary subcategories utilized by the authors?

14. List two behavioral patterns that people use to define relationships and control the exchange system.

15. List some of the emotions combined under the term *guilt*.

**Suggested
Readings**

Ackerman, N. *Psychodynamics of family life: Diagnosis and treatment in family relationships*. New York: Basic Books, 1958.

Bennet, E. *C. G. Jung*. New York: E. P. Dutton, 1962.

Bowen, M. Family psychotherapy, *American Journal of Orthopsychiatry*, 1961, *31*, 40–60.

Lidz, T. *The person*. New York: Basic Books, 1968.

Murphy, G. *Personality: A biosocial approach to origins and structure*. New York: Basic Books, 1966.

Sullivan, H. *The interpersonal theory of psychiatry*. New York: W. W. Norton, 1953.

7 Roles and Counterroles within the Family

All households have children or are expected to, and one of the responsibilities of any household system is to train the children for effective participation in adult roles.

C. F. Hockett, 1973 (2)

Advantages of Biosocial Approach

In man, social systems are functions of interacting biologic systems. However, we, as humans, would not be capable of considering biologic systems without tools, language, and concept formations that are imposed on our biologic systems by social systems.

In the last six chapters, we have been developing a theoretical model in which man is conceptualized as a unique open system of dynamically organized information. In this open system there is a continual flow of information among its composite biologic subsystems and between the system as a whole and its environment.

In order for this biologic open system to develop properties recognizable as human, it must at some time interact with an environment containing one or more other humans, that is, cultural or social systems. The study of the interacting human biologic and social systems we have called *biosociology*. We have emphasized that human behavior is a function of biologic and social processes and, therefore, serves as a common focal point of the biologic and sociologic sciences as they address man.

Biosociology as a theoretical conceptual model offers a number of advantages over less flexible models:

1. We can easily translate existing theories of behavior into more simple language.

2. We can understand how the transmission of information affects the internal and external relationships of man.

3. We can allow for enormous diversification among individuals without resorting to stereotyped categories.

Using the model of information flow in open systems, we may view the human self as an open system, or data bank, which continually changes with the input of new data from inside and outside the individual (that is, information exchanges, past and present). One of the major sources of information exchange occurs during conversations among individuals.

As we study human behavior, we may be able to discern certain repetitive patterns of communication among given individuals. These patterns are associated with the roles and counterroles making up the individual's self system, or identity, at a given time. These communication patterns help the individual to harmonize or synchronize his behavior with that of his cultural system and to predict and control his relationships with significant others.

One of the chief functions of communication, then, is to attempt continually to synchronize the individual self system within the culture. In any social interaction, the data exchanged in some way stabilize or redefine relationships between or among the involved self systems.

In this chapter, we will focus on segments of conversation to emphasize more clearly and simply how self-validating roles and counterroles evolve within families. The reader must use imagination to fill in the intonations and nonverbals, and must allow various sets of information to interact with his or her own self-concept and memories of similar interchanges in his or her own experience. For this reason, the examples given will have a different meaning for each reader.

It is hoped that the vignettes will mirror some aspect of each reader's self or stored experience. You should continually scrutinize not only the data being transmitted but the effect the data has on your self system.

Biasing Information   Each person tries to bias information in order to manipulate situations to benefit his own self concept. All of us do this. We may wish to deny that we do so because we may think that manipulation of behavior is bad or unfair. The following segment of conversation is illustrative of an attempt to define roles by biasing information. The mother is speaking to the father in the presence of Billy, their young son.

I want to talk to you about some things. . . . I'm afraid Billy is getting upset. . . . When we have our disagreements you have to keep your voice down because children don't understand. . . . I don't think it matters if he is hearing what we're saying now. We're talking like two civilized people but when you bellow like you did last night—. . . Billy, why don't you go play while Daddy and I talk? . . . Well, okay, you can stay here if you like. . . . He's such an affectionate child and so sensitive. Today I was talking to Mother and she was asking how we're getting along and I told her okay but I got a little emotional and I couldn't keep back the tears. Well, Billy sensed it right away and he put his arm around me and told me not to cry. And he said the cutest thing. You know what he said? . . . He said, "When I grow up I'm going to take care of Mommy and she won't cry anymore." . . . Now don't act so disgusted. You know I haven't been feeling well lately. Dr. Thomas says that I could have a thyroid problem and he thinks B-12 might help but he says he feels it could be my nerves. He's a very understanding man. Maybe Billy will grow up to be a doctor. How about that, Billy? Today he was really good when I got the headache. He brought me a damp cloth from the bathroom and put it over my eyes while I was lying down. Didn't you Billy? He's a very sensitive child and he worries a lot. He asked me while I was lying down, "You're not going to die, are you?" And I told him that I would die sometime but for him not to worry. I believe in being honest with children. . . . Why are you getting another beer? We never have a quiet conversation with each other. You're either losing your temper or drinking. I don't think that's a very good example for Billy. . . . When you grow up, you're not going to drink, are you, Billy? Drinking makes Mommy unhappy. . . . Well go ahead and if you insist on drinking, Billy and I will have to get along without you. . . . Well, go ahead and read your paper. Someday you'll be sorry you didn't give Billy more attention. Come on, Billy we'll look at your picture books. Don't bother Daddy. You know how he is when he's drinking. . . . No, I don't think you should go out and play with those children. They're too rough and besides, you'd get all dirty. Let me read you a story. How about *Jack and the Beanstalk*? You know, the one where the big giant chases the little boy?

In the preceding example, each family member continually scans the data to synchronize it with his or her own self system. The mother attempts to control the quantity and quality of information in order to make subsequent exchanges more predictable and favorable to herself. She struggles to obtain attention from her husband and son by communication techniques that may evoke guilt in her listeners. She also utilizes a process called *triangulation* which we will describe later.

Billy's self system is beginning to form as he listens to the conversation of his mother and father and watches the nonverbals of both parents. He is beginning to develop embryonic communication patterns. He is incorporating into his self system the expectations accompanying various roles including son, mother, father, male, female, child, and adult. He is beginning to individuate.

We might state metaphorically that the individual is a transient crystallization that emerges periodically from the group solution. The primary "group solution" is generally the family from which the individual evolves. As the individual self system develops, it constantly shifts and emits new data. Each new behavioral output is tested to see if the social system will validate it as being within the acceptable boundaries of the group self system. The conglomeration of self systems within a family reinforces and extinguishes patterns of behavior in a way similar to the paradigm of operant conditioning. The emerging individual self system, such as Billy's, exists largely in terms of what significant others in his family and limited social system think or have thought.

Communicating Frustration

While Billy's mother may seem to be a vicious individual who is making impossible demands upon her husband and raising a child who is programmed for problems, those more experienced in behavioral dynamics would begin to question the behavioral patterns in the family that have elicited her actions. What is the role of Billy's father in this particular family system? Perhaps it would be productive to hear his side of the story in this struggle for control. Consider the following scene as Billy's father returns from work and contributes to the family data pool.

Hi. How's everything? Billy okay? . . . How long 'til supper?
. . . Good! I'll have time for a martini. . . . So? Look, a lot of
men drink martinis for lunch. You know how uptight I get at the
office. If I can't let down here, where the hell am I supposed to
relax? . . . Had you rather I had gone out with the boys? Maybe
I should stop off at a tavern. It's just that I happen to like my
own home and besides it's a helluva lot cheaper this way. . . .
Now that's a lot of crap. You have not seen me really out of it
for several months. . . . So I tie one on every now and then. I

don't think it has a damn thing to do with my health. . . . No, starting the charcoal is too much trouble. Go ahead and put it in the oven. . . . Now look. What's buggin' you tonight? If anything, alcohol would make me want to charcoal the steak. Nothing makes charcoal taste better than gin. . . . Well, I can go on a diet and whip that off in no time. That's actually the reason I drink martinis. It avoids calories in a mix. . . . Well, who the hell likes gin and soda? I mean, for God's sake. Can you imagine what that shit would taste like? . . . What do you mean, watch my language? Billy will probably read worse words in the kindergarten bathroom. . . . No, this is only my second one, but if you keep up that tone of voice I will have another. As a matter of fact, I don't care if I do, do, do. . . . Why don't you tell your Mommy about it and she could come over and say "Naughty, naughty," to me. What a bitch! . . . No, I wasn't talking about you. I was talking about your dear mother. You're getting paranoid. What's the matter? Are you having your period or something or are you beginning a twenty year menopause? . . . Now don't start your wounded fawn routine. I know how you work hard. I know Billy is sensitive. I know the traffic is terrible. I know you don't get any cooperation at home. . . . I know, I know, I know. . . . I've already told you that you could hire a maid to come in and push your buttons. . . . My secretary works all day at the office and then goes home to take care of a house, a no-good husband and three kids. . . . Because I don't want to marry my secretary. I don't even want to screw my secretary. . . . Hell, he can't hear. He's in the bathroom and so what if—Great God, look at that smoke! Is it on fire? . . . You mean you haven't even turned it over? Oh, hell, you know I don't like it well done, much less overdone. Well, you got your charcoal. The whole damn house has been charcoaled. I hope the neighbors don't turn in a fire alarm. Are you sure *you* haven't been drinking? . . . Oh, forget it. You're right. I should be on a diet anyway. I'll tell you what. Why don't you call Billy and feed him? I need time to finish my drink and relax a bit more. . . . Look, four of these glasses would only make two large doubles. What's wrong with a couple of martinis before supper? You remember your father? He was a teetotaler and he's already dead. . . . You're right. I'm sorry. But he has been dead several years. . . . Maybe it just seems longer now that your mother is at large. Hey, that's good. At large, your mother—large. Get it? . . . Okay, okay. I know you don't talk about my parents. As a matter of fact, you rarely talk to my parents. . . . Well, somebody has to look in on them occasionally. After all, right after we were married I don't know what we would have done without them. So, let's not go through my dependency bit again. Granted I stop by to see Mom a few times a week, but I don't call her every day and she doesn't come and sit for hours. All in all, I'll bet you spend a lot more time with your mother than I do with mine. . . . You're right, it does sound a bit childish. Let's drop it. Did you hear

who won the ball game today? . . . Well, you're not too busy to
see "My Secret Sex Life" or whatever they call that washboard
weeper. Sometimes I wonder if women don't sit around and
masturbate while they watch those things. New, all improved
Zap makes a killing off of hiring a few hysterics and queers to
flit around in front of a TV camera with an organ playing in the
background. "Can Hannah Snodgrass find true happiness
shoveling horse manure at Belmont Race Track?" . . . I don't think
I was vulgar. Just because Billy laughed. That doesn't always
mean things are vulgar. Right, Billy? Besides, you must recall I
said manure. Perhaps I should have said organic matter, but you
must admit it could have been worse. . . . Oh, that. Well, next
time I will say fairy. You see, Billy, there are good fairies and
bad fairies, but all fairies have a thing about wands. . . . Okay,
okay. I guess I may as well empty the pitcher. No use in
cluttering the refrigerator with that little bit of martini. . . .
So, what's a half pint of gin? . . . Okay, a half-fifth of gin.
Tomorrow is Saturday and I don't have to go to the office until
late, so what the hades. Why not let it all hang out? . . . Yes, I do
have to go to the office and no, I do not care to pull tiny weeds
away from whiney, smog-laden flowers. Live and let live. That's
my motto. Anything that can survive in this polluted world
deserves its chance to be miserable. . . . Let's turn on the TV
and watch some wholesome all-American family in which mother
and brood in their cozy suburban nest, hereafter referred to as
trap, humiliate and degrade a wretched piece of protoplasm
commonly known as Dad. Talk about violence. God! . . . No, I can't
think of any other place I would rather be. In fact, I can't really
think of anything any more. That's why I called it a trap. . . . No,
I'm kidding. I mean, it's great. Really. One has to deteriorate
sometime. There's no escaping that, so why not do it gracefully
in a little white casket with green shutters and a two car garage.
Everyone else does. Why fight it? Besides, I haven't given up the
possibility of living vicariously through Billy. Someday my son
may become vice-president of a huge corporation and be able
to afford a large brick casket on a corner lot and then I can
shuffle slowly out of my smaller casket and buttonhole passers-by
like the ancient mariner. Then with boney finger I shall point to
the largest sarcophagus in the adjoining subdivision and with
cracking voice cry, "That's my boy." God, what fun. I can't wait.
. . . You're right, you're right. I am being sarcastic. Please
excuse me. I have no right to take out my frustrations from a
hard day at the office on the greatest little family in the world.
Billy, you understand your old Dad was just kidding, don't
you? . . . Good, good. Would you hand me that stock market
report there? . . . Thanks. Must keep up with the important things in
life. . . . No, thanks, honey. I'm really not hungry. I'll make myself a
sandwich later. No, really, honestly. Thanks anyway.

What? . . . Oh, sure, sure, no, the TV won't bother me a bit.

Huh? What? Oh, is it that time already? I must have dropped off. Is Billy in bed already? . . . No, I was not in an alcoholic stupor. I was tired. This has been a rough week. You just can't seem to understand that, can you? Someone must work so that others may live. Want to watch the late show? . . . It's a western with Gary Cooper. The nice thing about westerns—men seemed to be men—probably because there were fewer women around out there . . . I never tried kissing a horse, but there might be some advantages. I never saw a horse with rollers in its hair. Why do you have to wear those things anyway? . . . Nothing sexier than a woman in her housecoat with grease on her face, rollers in her hair, sitting on a commode, smoking a cigarette and reading a magazine about Hollywood marriages. God! . . . No, I wasn't referring to you. I was merely free associating. I swear there was absolutely nothing personal about it. . . . Well, offhand, I can't remember you making me feel like a stud horse lately. . . . Skip it. Do you want to watch this flick? . . . Okay. I think I've seen it anyway. I'll be up in a few minutes, as soon as I see how it opens. . . . Say, you know, that's not really a bad movie. I think we saw it right after we were married. . . . Are you asleep? Are you asleep already? Oh, crap."

Billy's father expresses his frustration (hostility) about the lack of control he has on the family information-exchange system through the use of several communication techniques. The most obvious is sarcastic humor. He implies he is unappreciated for his hard work thereby evoking guilt in his wife. In order to bolster his self system he derogates his wife's behavioral patterns. He explains his deficits in meeting his own expectations by blaming the expectations of the family as being responsible for his frustrations. He attempts to control the way that relationships are defined by emphasizing the magnitude of his sacrifice. He, too, utilizes triangulation in his reference to his wife's mother and to his secretary. He avoids any expectations from his wife concerning his sexual prowessness by drinking and staying up after she goes to bed. By communicating disgust that she is already asleep, he may disguise any doubts he may have concerning his role as a male sexual partner. Evidence of frustration or hostility in communication patterns often stems from insecurity and may be considered as an abstract fight–flight pattern.

Competition for Control of the Family System

Persons involved in family units are always competing for control. It is seldom that one individual controls the entire family system at all times. Control shifts as family constellations shift and as children mature and copy the behavioral patterns of their parents and other individuals within their social systems. Adolescents begin to learn control techniques of their own and set priorities as they search for synchronization within the family group. So-called "normal" adolescent behavior is characterized by the quest for identity and control as illustrated in the following vignette, in which Billy, now in his teens, is making a request.

> Hey, Mom, can I have the car for a couple of hours? . . . I just want to go over to Butch's for a while. . . . Because we're working on that ham radio set I told you and Dad about. . . . I know it's four o'clock but we never have supper 'til after six anyway. . . . But I don't want to stop at the grocery store. . . . Why can't Dad pick that stuff up on his way home from work? . . . I know he's tired, but hell. . . . Okay, okay. . . . Damn. There must be 25 things on this list. . . . It's not disrespectful; everybody says hell and damn. . . . Okay, I'm sorry. . . . Now can I have the car? . . . Drop granny off at Aunt Maudies? Ah, hell, why can't the old bag take a taxi? . . . I know she's over 80 and we're not going to have her with us much longer, but why does she have to spend her last days with me? . . . Yeah, I love her but who wants to drive all over town with a gray-haired old crock? . . . Oh, shit, forget it. I didn't want the car anyway.

Billy's relinquishment of his request for the family automobile is an acceptance of transient situational control by his mother. His priorities have been set to adjust to his own limitations—it is easier to give up the car than to meet all the expectations required to get it. However, he defies his mother's total control and differentiates himself from her by the continued use of already forbidden profanity and vulgarities.

Security and Acceptance

The security of the self system depends on acceptance of its behavioral patterns by the group self. Patterns of behavior become a part of the individual's self system conditioned by group acceptance. This acceptance as a reinforcement need not always be constant. Psychological experiments in conditioned behavior indicate that intermittent reinforcement makes conditioned patterns more difficult to extinguish than constant reinforcement followed by constant lack of reinforcement.

The security of Billy's self system is dependent on his relinquishing his present request in the face of his mother's opposition, an opposition which is manifested by the addition of so many expectations contingent on the use of the car that Billy's acceptance of her role definition would be a compromise of the integrity of his self system.

Adolescence is a time for testing many behavioral patterns in the struggle for control and the bid for attention. The information exchange system is in a constant state of flux as parents try to reinforce or extinguish data emitted by the adolescent. Attempts to maintain a synchronized family self system may be frustrating to all family members.

Adolescents use various communication techniques in an effort to share in the definition of relationships. We have considered the birth of the self system as analogous to parturition. If we continue the analogy, the period of adolescence might be likened to the cutting of the umbilical cord. The self system of the adolescent can now survive separately from its mother although it is often influenced by parental positive and negative reinforcement patterns.

Adding Members to a Family System

No family or social unit is continually free of dissynchrony, but it usually operates at a functional level even though placed under stress by the fluid nature of relationships. A stressful situation for any family is the addition of another member to the group, whether it be a sibling or an older relative.

Older persons (usually grandparents) may come to live in a family unit about the time their grandchildren are attempting to reify their self systems and establish their own control techniques. The parents of the adolescents (who are also the offspring of grandparents) are sometimes caught in the middle of a multigenerational struggle for control. All individuals in this shifting multigenerational family are then confronted with the task of renegotiating how their relationships are defined with each other.

This can be illustrated by the following dialogue:

MOTHER: I never should have given up my farm; I'm just a bother to you.

DAUGHTER: Oh, Mother, we love having you. Don't pay any attention to Harry. He doesn't mean what he says.

MOTHER: I made a mistake when I sold the farm and moved into your house. You all used to enjoy visiting there. Billy played with the dog and Harry went fishing in the pond. But I thought if I sold the farm I could help send Billy to college. I haven't got many years left and I don't need the money.

DAUGHTER: Now, Mother, we've been through that a hundred times. You know you couldn't manage that farm with your arthritis. It's not the money. I worried about you being there alone. What if you had fallen and broken a hip while you were out feeding the chickens? It might have been hours before anyone found you.

MOTHER: I sold the chickens right after your father died, all but three hens and a rooster, and I could feed them from the back porch.

DAUGHTER: But you know how you worried about the pastures growing up. And Harry doesn't have time to supervise hired help to run the farm and keep up his law practice here in town. Besides, we like to have you near us.

MOTHER: You're just saying that to make me feel good. I know when I'm a burden. I don't think Billy likes me, either.

DAUGHTER: Of course he does, Mother; he used to beg to visit Grandmother.

MOTHER: Then why does he play his records so loud? He knows it get on my nerves. I've asked him to turn it down but he turns it off and gets in such a huff. When he turns it on again, it's just as loud as before.

DAUGHTER: I'll have Harry speak to him about it. I'm sure he won't mind.

MOTHER: Maybe you'd better not! I'm afraid Harry is angry at me, too.

DAUGHTER: Now, Mother, don't be silly. Why should Harry be angry with you?

MOTHER: Well, last night when I told him that the late TV show he was watching was keeping me awake, he looked angry.

DAUGHTER: Oh, he was just tired. You know how he is when he gets tired.

MOTHER: Why should he be tired? All he did yesterday afternoon was sit around in Doctor Green's waiting room while I was waiting to see the doctor.

DAUGHTER: Well, doctors make him nervous. You know how men are.

MOTHER: I'm just a burden. Everyone would be better off if I was dead.

DAUGHTER: Mother, stop that.... Say, where's Billy? He's been home from school over fifteen minutes and I haven't heard a peep from him. Maybe I'd better go check on him.

[While her daughter is out of the room, Grandmother quietly moves Harry's favorite chair away from the television set.]

DAUGHTER: Mother! Come here, quick! Billy has taken some of your pain pills!

[Grandmother grabs the small bottle and begins to check the contents as daughter wrings her hands.]

MOTHER: Well, he must have taken at least three of my pills.

DAUGHTER: Mother, we'd better get him to the hospital; I'll call Harry.

MOTHER: Billy, how *could* you take my pills? What if I don't have enough to last me until my next appointment with Doctor Green?

The parent of an adolescent who also has a parent living in the same family unit is frequently required to switch roles and redefine relationships, depending upon the nature of the information exchanged and the circumstances surrounding the interchange. Adolescents and older individuals may be equally narcissistic (self-centered) in demanding attention to all their respective needs, increasing competition within the family.

In the example just given, Billy's mother is torn among her roles of mother, child, and wife. The grandmother senses that her roles are of decreasing value to the family exchange system. This insecurity results in her attempting to regain some control by evoking guilt in her child. If Billy's mother responds by giving attention to her mother this may produce insecurity in Billy so that he has to exhibit behavior that will draw attention to him (for example, by taking pills).

The shift in this nuclear family by the addition of a new member has led to difficulty in predicting the information that will be shared. The lack of predictability leads to insecurity and masked fight–flight patterns. The aggression in these patterns is disguised by pseudoaltruism, that is, information that one or more of the family members are making sacrifices out of their love for other members. The anger is verbalized as "I am suffering for your sake." This statement implies "You owe me something" or "I expect something from you but since I am suffering you should not expect anything from me."

This mixture of disclaimed anger or aggression with verbalized signals of affection evokes a similar mixture of ambivalent feelings in others within the family. We have termed these feelings "guilt." Since most individuals find guilt an uncomfortable feeling, they attempt to avoid it or retaliate with similar communication patterns. The use of guilt in the power struggle to define relationships, control information, and obtain attention for their threatened self systems is evident in the multigenerational struggle portrayed in the previous dialogue.

Human Behavioral Patterns Colored by Digital Operation

Certain patterns of behavior arising from the analogic processes (for example, mating, mothering, feeding, avoidance of dangerous situations) are markedly colored and embellished by the human digital operation. This peculiarly human function has been evident in each of the vignettes we have studied thus far. Cultural systems have digitalized these patterns into role stereotypes ("A good mother is . . ." "A husband should . . .") of an individual's self system. These stereotypes do not seem prominent in nonhuman animals. A female opossum may mother her young, but we would not expect her to be capable of digitalizing this process into a verbal abstraction, "I am a mother" and to further digitalize by stating, "I am a good mother because I do for my offspring what opossums who live in my area prescribe."

We can accept that a mother opossum might appear anxious on weaning her young but it is doubtful that she would appear guilty about not being a good mother and threaten suicide if the young opossums neglected to give her attention throughout their lives. Nor do young opossums show any indication of guilt if they do not care for their aging mothers. These patterns of behavior are most prominent in the human animal and are dependent on digital operations in which the role of mother has been incorporated into self systems.

Since opossums are incapable of digitalized abstractions, they are unable to engage in those cultural processes, that is language and self-differentiation, which dominate human society. Without these cultural tools, opossums are precluded from complex communication patterns among several individuals. A prominent human communication pattern of this nature involving three or more individuals is called triangulation.

Triangulation

Triangulation can be defined as a communication technique used by one member of a group to obtain attention and shift responsibility and unwanted expectations away from himself by communicating to another member about a third member. By using this technique, or communication pattern, the individual attempts to control information exchange systems and insure self-validating responses to his or her behaviors. Triangulation is evident in some of the preceding vignettes.

A thorough discussion of the nature of family triangles is given in the book *Family interaction: A dialogue between family researchers and family therapists*, edited by

James L. Framo. One of the contributing authors who chose to remain anonymous wrote,

A system larger than three persons becomes a series of interlocking triangles. The following are some of the characteristics of functioning of a single triangle. As tension mounts in a two-person system, it is usual for one to be more uncomfortable than the other, and for the uncomfortable one to 'triangle in' a third person by telling the second person a story about the triangled one. This relieves the tension between the first two, and shifts the tension between the second and third [1, pp. 123–124]

The following vignette illustrates triangulation as Billy's grandmother continues her attempts to gain attention and to control the family by shifting the blame for her decisions or lack of decision on Harry's relationship with Aunt Virgie in order to relieve the rising tensions between her own self system and that of her daughter. The triangulation is coupled with somatic complaints to further decrease the grandmother's responsibility for meeting expectations. Guilt is a prominent characteristic of this type of interchange.

DAUGHTER: Mother, it's such a beautiful afternoon, Harry and I are going for a drive out in the country and we want you to come along.

MOTHER: Well, Alice, that's sweet of you, honey, but I think maybe I'd better just stay here. I don't feel like getting dressed up.

DAUGHTER: Mother, you don't have to dress up to sit in the car and you're always saying you never do anything but just sit in the house and watch television.

MOTHER: What if we had an accident? I wouldn't want to have my old clothes on if we had to go to a hospital. And there's so many cars on the roads these days.

DAUGHTER: There is a lot of traffic and I know you get nervous. Well, then, let's go visit Aunt Virgie. It's been quite a while since you've seen her and you were saying the other day how you'd like to go over there.

MOTHER: That would be nice, Alice, but Harry doesn't like Virgie. He never has liked her since we had that quarrel over your father's will. And I get uncomfortable when they're in the same room.

DAUGHTER: Mother, that's all in your imagination. That little mix-up over Dad's will was settled years ago. But if it's going to worry you, Harry can stay home this afternoon and watch the baseball game and we'll go.

MOTHER: Now, Alice. I know you're trying to be sweet but you and Harry go ahead and do something together. You need to get away from me for a while, anyway, and just be alone. Besides I'm used to being by myself, and I don't mind any more. Except when you're out late at night.

DAUGHTER: Mother, we hardly ever go out at night. But let's not get into that now. Please come and go with me; it'll be good for you to get out.

MOTHER: Honey, I'd really like to, but my feet swell in the afternoons and my good shoes are too tight.

DAUGHTER: Oh, Mother, sometimes you can get so difficult. It's your own fault you never get to go anywhere. You always have a dozen excuses for everything.

MOTHER: Alice, dear, now you're angry with me, aren't you? I guess I should have told you the truth from the beginning. I've been having these bad chest pains since early this morning.

DAUGHTER: Mother, why didn't you say so? You should be in bed right now. I'll go call Dr. Green and ask him what to do. I'm sorry I lost my temper. I didn't know you were feeling badly.

MOTHER: I understand dear. I should have said something sooner, but I hate to worry you. Would you mind asking Harry to keep the television turned down? Maybe I'd better try to sleep a little.

The use of somatic complaints is a common communication technique for controlling the information exchange, shifting responsibility to others, and decreasing expectations from others. It is especially effective if the complaints imply a life-threatening illness. By contributing these data to the information pool, the individual forces significant others to suppress further any expression of hostility and to increase the amount of attention they give their ailing loved one.

Since their behavior is motivated by guilt, their communication may occasionally appear stilted and insincere. This decreases the predictability of the information exchange, elevates anxiety, and results in more emphasis on somatic symptoms. Hypochondriasis is a communication technique that all of us will encounter many times. The frustration of families in responding to this type of information is frequently shared by the health professional.

Health professionals may reify the family triangle since each examination and each pill now validates that the suffering individual is not responsible. Attempts by a health professional to break this pattern may result in an increased insecurity since the entire family may utilize the sick role of an individual as a focal point for deficits in their information pool.

The daughter may lower the expectations on her self system by stating, "I would like to do more but I am worried about mother." The husband and son can enjoy an uneasy truce built around not upsetting the suffering grandmother or mother who is suffering because grandmother is suffering.

Complexity of Family Systems

It is prudent to be aware of the complexity of interlocking family communication patterns before attempting to eradicate what may initially seem to be the problem as indicated by complaints of various family members. These complaints may be a synchronizing factor in the family's information exchange system. Unless other techniques for synchrony can be put in their place, the removal of complaints may result in chaos within the family, and a frantic search by family members for another method of synchronization. We will address patterns used in attempting to synchronize individual and group behavior in subsequent chapters.

The hunger for information and the search for synchrony makes us human. The tuning of the self is a life-long process. Avoidance of conflict requires continual synchronizing or tuning of the individual self system with that of the family and community, and this tuning of social self systems with progressively larger conglomerates including national and international self systems. Tuning is dependent on communication, that is, synchronized data sharing among the arbitrary delineated units.

References

1. Framo, J. (Ed.). *Family interaction: A dialogue between family researchers and family therapists.* New York: Springer, 1972.

2. Hockett, C. *Man's place in nature.* New York: McGraw-Hill, 1973, p. 224.

Suggested Readings

Adler, A. *Social interest: A challenge to mankind.* New York: Capricorn Books, 1964.

Bandura, A., *Principles of behavior modification.* New York: Holt, Rinehart & Winston, 1969.

Berne, E. *Games people play: The psychology of human relationships*. New York: Grove Press, 1964.

Bowan, M. Family psychotherapy. *American Journal of Orthopsychiatry, 1961, 31*, 40–60.

Bowlby, J. *Maternal care and mental health*. New York: Schocken Books, 1966.

Fleck, S. Family dynamics and origin of schizophrenia. *Psychosomatic Medicine*, 1960, *22*, 333–334.

Freud, S. The ego and the superego. In T. Parsons, E. Shils, K. Naegele, and J. Pitts (Eds.), *Theories of society: Foundations of modern sociological theory*, Vol. II. New York: Free Press, 1961.

Haley, J. *Strategies of psychotherapy*. New York: Grune & Stratton, 1963.

Kessler, J. *Psychopathology of childhood*. Englewood Cliffs, New Jersey: Prentice-Hall, 1966.

Mead, G. Taking the role of the other. In T. Parsons, E. Shils, K. Naegele, and J. Pitts (Eds.), *Theories of society: Foundations of modern sociological theory*, Vol. II. New York: Free Press, 1961.

Mullahy, P. Harry Stack Sullivan. In A. Freedman, H. Kaplan, and B. Sadock (Eds.), *Comprehensive textbook of psychiatry/II*, Vol. II. Baltimore: Williams & Wilkins, 1975.

Rank, O. *The trauma of birth*. New York: Harcourt, Brace, 1929.

Ruesch, J. Communication and psychiatry. In A. Freedman, H. Kaplan, and B. Sadock (Eds.), *Comprehensive Textbook of Psychiatry/II*, Vol. I. Baltimore: Williams & Wilkins, 1975.

Satir, V. *Conjoint family therapy*. Palo Alto, California: Science and Behavior Books, 1967.

Shamsie, S. (Ed.). *Youth: Problems and approaches*. Philadelphia, Pennsylvania: Lea & Febiger, 1972.

Skinner, B. *Beyond freedom and dignity*. New York: Bantam/Vintage Books, 1971.

Spradlin, W. Family roles of the elderly as a focus in teaching comprehensive medicine, *The Journal of Medical Education, 1967, 42* (11), Pp. 1045–1048.

Sullivan, H. *The interpersonal theory of psychiatry*. New York: Norton, 1953.

Thomas, W. *The family constellation: Its effects on personality and social behavior*. New York: Springer, 1969.

Watson, J. *Behaviorism*. New York: Norton, 1924.

Wolpe, J. The behavior therapy approach. In S. Arieti (Ed.), *American Handbook of Psychiatry*, Vol. I. New York: Basic Books, 1974.

Suggested Questions

1. Give three advantages of biosociology as a theoretical conceptual model.

2. Give one of the chief functions of communication.

3. Why would an individual try to bias information?

4. Discuss some of the communication techniques Billy's father uses to express his frustration.

5. Give one characteristic of "normal" adolescent behavior.

6. On what does the security of the self system depend?

7. Discuss the task confronting those individuals in a shifting multigeneration family.

8. What colors certain human behavioral patterns arising from the analogic processes?

9. Give a definition of triangulation.

10. Discuss the use of somatic complaints as a communication technique.

11. Why is it prudent to be aware of the complexity of interlocking family communication patterns before attempting to eradicate what may initially seem to be "the problem?"

12. What does avoidance of conflict require?

8 Stress and Life Styles

When mathematics and chemistry define your world, it has no meaning; the world dries up. But, for you, as you walk the streets, engage others, live your life, your world is charged with meaning, filled with purposes, conflicted or aligned, at every level.

Arthur Deikman, 1976(1)

Man as a Biologic System

We have postulated that man is a biologic system and, therefore, that all of his behavior must have a biologic base. We have also postulated that human behavior is the product of social systems. There is the temptation to be drawn into the unproductive debate of whether a given behavior originates more from the biologic or the social factors making up a given individual. One might just as well ask whether sodium atoms or chloride atoms are responsible for the crystalline properties of salt. Without either set of atoms, the relationship among all the atoms would not be the same, and the crystalline properties of table salt would not be present.

We cannot dissect out either biologic or sociologic factors from human behavior and still be studying human behavior. Therefore, the following definition is worth repeating. *Human behavior may be defined as a function of all of the dynamic biosocial processes that interact in the system of relationships we call man.*

This does not mean that we cannot study the behavioral effect of shifting the human biologic substrate or altering the social environment; many of these rearrangements will be associated with behavioral changes. It would be oversimplifying matters to assume that since changes arise from biologic or biochemical alteration, biologic factors are the cause of certain behaviors. Nor can we state that social factors are responsible for any given patterns of behavior, even though a shift in social milieu may alter the behavior. We belabor the point because, in our experience, students of behavior often fall into the antinomy of viewing human behavior as an either–or phenomenon.

Life Styles   In studying human behavior we note that each individual is different from any other. Each self system is unique. It would be easier to dismiss the individual self phenomenon as a myth and to proceed with the rapidly advancing neurochemical, pharmacologic, and neurophysiologic studies, hoping that when enough is known in these fields that the "self" will fall into place. This may be the case eventually. Certainly, many students of behavior who have addressed the problem of "self" have bogged down in philosophic and epistomologic tautologies. And yet, we constantly hear and use phrases like *low self-esteem*, *self-consciousness,* and *insecure self-concepts.* The self must then be treated as an entity. The "me" or the "I" is the central reference point of perceptive organization and communication.

What is the me or the I? I look at my finger and "It is my finger," as though it were apart from me, a possession of me. I wish it to move and it does, but not in response to vocal request. If I had the perceptive equipment to visualize the sodium, potassium, and other ions rushing about in my body, I might command them, using the code of interpersonal communication, to enter my neurons or not to enter my neurons and it would probably have little effect on whether they did or not. And yet, without hesitation, I accept the finger, the neurons, and the sodium, potassium, and other ions as mine. What, then, is the me apart from these components? The impasse seems to stem from our conditioned pattern of referring to the digitally coded data concerning our bodies, thoughts, and feelings as the "me." The other codes, including those of the ions, fluids, and cells of our body, are as much the me as the digital code involved in speech. However, by our digital operation we conceptualize our parts as differentiated from the coded data we call me.

This coded data called the me or self system, is utilized in the process termed *reflective consciousness.* By this process I am aware of my "self." Our digital operation is continually exchanging information with other code systems within our bodies but not via the language that we use in interpersonal communication. We often single out the data coding process that is amenable to pairing with language and term it our "self," our "me," our "I." This verbal representation distorts by oversimplification but use of the self referencing apparatus has allowed humans to (a) expand relationships with other humans (b) become free of total dependency on genetic programming and stimulus locked experiential learning, and (c) vastly increase their information pool. To designate this digitalized code as the "me" is a useful working abstraction.

Whether we call the self system an illusion, a myth, or the goal of the universe, this empirical delineation or subject–object dichotomy is the product and producer of the cultural activity we term *civilization*. And it influences all human behaviors.

Just as each individual's behavior is different, each person's present behavior differs continually from his past behavior. However, there is enough repetition in his behavioral patterns so that we may recognize him. These recurrent patterns, which we will call a *life style*, influence the way in which the individual fulfills the various roles included in his or her self system.

A person's life style can be defined, then, as the behavioral patterns repeatedly used by an individual in developing and maintaining the shifting roles of his self system. These life style patterns are evidenced in the behaviors each of us exhibits in day-to-day living, and influence our self-concepts and the way others respond to us. If the response of others is predictable, it reinforces our life style.

Each individual self-concept differs in the number and type of roles incorporated. Each role is different, depending on the life style of the individual fulfilling the role. This, in turn, is dependent on the function of the biosocial subsystems composing the individual. This flexibility makes each individual unique and different, even if he or she adopts socially stereotyped roles in his or her self-concept.

For example, one individual may appear to be quite sociable, coming into contact with many other people each day, whereas another person may appear to be quite secluded, hardly leaving the house. The first might be said to be leading an *extroverted* life style while the second might be said to be leading an *introverted* life style. Yet both persons might be incorporating the same social role (for example, mother) in their self-concepts.

One mother of several children may see herself as an outgoing person who needs a lot of stimulation to function well in her role as mother, so she may be active in the local PTA, a garden club, politics, and church activities. Her idea of motherhood includes all these functions. Her way of life is her life style. Another mother of several children might be quite introverted and not wish to be with other people, but choose to stay at home and become an expert cook and decorator, spending many hours on her home. Her interpretation of the role of mother and the activities she enjoys in that role make up her life style.

Search for Autonomy

The particular life style we adopt gives us the illusion of autonomy. As we build more and more of a structure around us that we can call exclusively ours, we begin to think of our self systems in even more concrete terms. We live as if our self systems were entities, things that we must protect and defend and that we must keep in harmony or in tune with our social systems.

In our search for the answers to make our self systems or self-concepts synchronous and to tune ourselves with others around us, we are so innovative and versatile that no two people are alike. When you perceive that another person is "like" yourself, the conceptualizing process is similar to looking in a mirror and momentarily seeing yourself reflected there. The reflection is transient, as any two individuals who marry because they appear alike soon discover.

This point may seem obvious, but it is more complicated than we first realize. We choose our marriage partners, our friends, and our social groups and give reasons for our choices such as, "He and I are alike," "All the people in my crowd think alike," "We all like to do the same things." These similarities in taste are often quite superficial. People who have been friends for years will decide to become roommates and then find themselves differing on so many seemingly trivial points (such as whether or not to leave the cap on the tube of toothpaste) that they may become disenchanted with the friendship and say something like, "I never really knew

Bill. I thought I knew him, but then I started living with him. He's nothing like you think he is."

The small adjustments in living that each person makes and that contribute to his or her life style are important because they add to our illusion of autonomy. It is probably not possible to find two people who have life styles so similar that they do not, at least occasionally, clash or fall into disagreement. Each of us is continually trying to stay in harmony or synchronous with our environment. These efforts result in our having to make changes in our self system.

Shifts in Self-Concept

We use various adaptational mechanisms to maintain a more or less stable relationship to society. These adaptational mechanisms have to be adjusted constantly in order to sustain our self-concepts. Most of these adjustments are functional, and allow us enormous flexibility in patterns of living and coding information. The shifts we make are so slight or so smoothly accomplished that we sometimes are not even aware we are making them.

All of us are under stress. The occurrence of stress situations is frequent in the life span of each individual. People who claim that they have no problems or are never under stress are either (*a*) refusing to acknowledge or recognize stressful situations, or (*b*) have developed attitudinal sets that allow them to make "fine tuning" moves in their lives so that the problems never develop to the point where they result in feelings of being out of control.

Adjustments to Stress

Crises may occur when we are *forced* to make a shift in self-concept. Examples of these shifts are seen in puberty, adulthood, marriage, parenthood, and occasionally with changing educational and employment status. The earlier crises usually occur when the individual self system is relatively flexible and multipotential. This type of flexibility may produce the restless insecurity often seen in the adolescent who has not yet acquired sufficient information to choose a life style. It is during this rather frightening period that the adolescent may shift rapidly in processing information, changing direction repeatedly. Because of a lack of stability in their early family systems, some individuals exhibit these adolescent-like searching behaviors throughout their lifetimes, never being able to adopt stable behavioral constellations. Most of us do learn to adjust to stress and do become fairly stable in our patterns of relating to others.

Learning to Use Others

As we develop our life styles we are constantly in the process of using each other. This is sometimes difficult for students to understand because they have been led to believe that using another person is somehow bad or manipulative. However, we could not function without using each other. Teachers must use students in order to teach. Students could not be students in any organized educational system unless they used teachers. The "self" is in the process of either using or being used at almost any given time and its adroitness at this process makes it either functional or dysfunctional.

We use others to develop our patterns of relating emotionally. We sometimes use others as excuses for doing or not doing something. We like to believe that we are quite self-sufficient and that our behavioral paradigms are pure. An individual may say, "I do things this way because that's the way I am," or "I've been like this ever since I can remember." Yet, subsequent qualifying statements concerning his behavior indicate his dependency on the behavior of others and his use of other self-concepts. "I smoke because my parents smoked." Or "I don't smoke because my parents did and I want to be different." "We never had any liquor in our house so I never learned to drink." Or "My father and brother were both alcoholics, my husband is an alcoholic, so I drink too."

Similarities in behavioral patterns or life styles have led to elaborate classifications of personality types and character traits. These are described in most standard texts of psychology and psychiatry. These categories or classifications are working constructs and, although they do denote similarities, they differ among individuals and, from time to time, in the same individual.

Many times we will hear a person described as "paranoid" (suspicious) or "hysterical" (theatrical) and assume that our description is conveying something about that individual. These diagnostic labels and descriptive terms mean little unless we know the individual well enough to operationalize our definitions of paranoid or hysterical with reference to exhibited behaviors. Even standard texts will differ in their definitions with respect to many of the diagnostic entities thrown around so freely in our conversation.

All of us display, at some time in our lives, certain patterns of behavior that could be diagnosed "paranoid" or "hysterical," but diagnostic labels mean little except as a way of passing only the most general information about an individual's behavior on to another individual. Our patterns of behavior change, sometimes quite rapidly, depending on our circumstances, our states of arousal, and other variables.

Attempts to Maintain Integrity

Each individual attempts to adopt patterns of behavior that help to maintain a semblance of integrity for his particular self system and life style. Although those patterns of behavior may appear unacceptable to others and even to himself at times, once an individual has adopted a life style with which he feels comfortable, he is unlikely to make major changes unless compelled to do so. Rather than make major adjustments in his self system, the individual will develop *excuse clauses*, which can be utilized when he becomes miserable or reaches an impasse. Excuse clauses can be defined as the information that an individual utilizes in order to keep in tune with his information-exchange system and thus avoid intolerable discomfort.

Some of the excuse clauses we utilize to keep us in synchrony or in harmony with those around us are not necessarily beneficial to us. In fact, they may prevent the development of more responsive data-exchange systems. They do allow us to continue in a life style we find comfortable. For example, a shy individual who enters a large university town from a small high school may be overwhelmed by the large classes and the rather impersonal attitudes of his teachers and peers. The student may lack the necessary skills to become a part of the information-exchange system of a large college campus, and so withdraw even further and begin to fall behind. The student may then say, "The people here are unfriendly. The teachers take no interest in me. It is not my fault but theirs that I am flunking out of school." By arranging information in this way, the student can defend his or her self-concept and change to a smaller school or drop out of school altogether without losing face. This type of excuse clause maintains the integrity of the self system without requiring major adjustments in self-perception.

The primary function of an excuse clause, whatever its form, is to defend the self-concept against stress and thereby permit the person to continue in a particular life style.

**Escape Techniques
That Decrease
Tension**

The majority of people avoid major changes in their self concepts by participating in socially acceptable ways of sharing their excuse clauses. The excuse clauses that an individual utilizes are more effective when validated by others, especially significant others such as close friends and family members. Some persons are able to alleviate tension in their self systems by exchanging information with strangers. Perhaps this type of technique can best be illustrated by a vignette. The following conversation takes place in a bar, a relatively common place for this type of interchange.

Damned right! That Jerry West was the best damn basketball player in the leagues. . . . You notice what color he is, too. That's what's ruining basketball nowadays, they put all those Watusis on the teams, I mean, the games nowadays look like some sort of African rituals. . . . Let's have another one. . . . No, you bought the last one. Two more doubles with a little water on the side, bartender. I should have been home a half-hour ago, but, hell, a man has to blow off some steam sometimes. If the old lady's going to bitch about a half-hour, she may as well bitch about an hour. . . . Damn right. . . . I don't give a damn what these women's libbers say. It's the men that make the wheels turn in this country. It's men that fight to keep the world free. . . . Damn bunch of lesbians tryin' to stir up trouble. Women don't know what a good thing they got. I mean, seriously, what do men get out of marriage? Just a steady piece, right? . . . Have you ever stopped to think how much we men pay for all that? Hell, we could buy it off the street two or three times a week a lot cheaper than what we're payin' for it. And on top of that, we wouldn't have to put up with all that nagging and bitching. What this country needs is several million geisha girls. You know, like they have over in Japan. That would be livin', wouldn't it, yessir, man. Really livin'. . . . No, I wasn't in the service but I heard some of the guys who were over there talk about it. That must really be something. Layin' around in a hot bath gettin' rubbed down. Man, I would eat that with a spoon. . . . The trouble with women now is they don't know their place. They want us to wait on them. Ain't that a crock? Work hard all day and go home to listen to yak, yak. And you notice they never say anything. They can talk for a solid hour and never say nothin! I don't mean to say all women are like that. There are exceptions. You take my mother, for example. When my old man ran off, she went to work in a department store and raised us four kids. Now there was a woman for you, rest her soul. I always get a little choked up when I think about her. She worked like a dog for us. You know, she even wanted me to go to college but I went to work and helped out with the others. I was the oldest and I stayed there and helped support them until they were old enough to leave home. . . . Do you think they appreciate it? . . . Why, hell, no. I rarely ever see the bastards. My kid brother still owes me money. After I got married she lived with us until—she had a stroke. I'm sorry I got emotional but you know how it is. . . . Sure, I'll have another one with you. Thanks! Where you from? . . . I never been out there but with the kids in school, you know how it is. . . . Yeah, as soon as I get the kids off my back I'm going to try to save up and get me one of those camper deals and me and the old lady will drive all the way across and back. I planned to drive out to Indiana to visit an uncle last summer but my wife isn't well. Her organs fell down or something. You know women are always sick. Have you noticed that, too? . . . God, I hope this summer ain't as hot as last summer. My air conditioning unit broke down about the middle of July. I'm telling you it was hell. It rained a lot last summer, too. What with the humidity, I ain't kiddin', it was terrible. Last winter was bad, too. They really ought to do something about the snowplows in this city. . . . It was bad out there, too, huh? You know something; not to change the subject, but you're a likeable son-of-a-bitch. You really are. I mean, you really got a good head on your shoulders. Too many guys nowadays don't know their ass from a hole in the ground, but you got class. . . . Well, I try to keep up with things. I guess I do all right for a guy with not much education. At least I got common sense which is more than you can say about a lot of your educated eggheads. . . . Damn right. . . . God, look at the time. My old lady will kill me. Say, why don't we get together again for a drink? . . . No, I can't this week. I'm what you might call booked up. . . . Oh, just passing through, huh? That's a damn shame. I don't know when I've enjoyed myself more than talking with you this evening. If you're ever through this way again, look me up. I only live a few blocks from here. Almost everybody knows me. Just ask for Ralph. What did you say your name was? . . . Glad to meet you, Smith. That's an easy one to remember. Like I say, if you're through this way again, give me a ring, okay? Hang in there, Buddy. See you around.

The advantages to the speaker in the above vignette are those of anonymity with low levels of expectation and responsibility. Ralph is using the tension-reducing technique of venting his feelings to a stranger and allowing himself the luxury of saying things which he probably would not say to significant others in his information-exchange system. He is giving himself the illusion of talking to a person who "understands" him and will not have to put this illusion to the test of reality.

Ralph's excuse clauses include the blaming of minority groups (females, blacks), his unappreciative relatives, the weather, his wife's illness, social classes, finances, technology (broken air conditioner), for dissynchrony between his life style and his self system. He precludes any validation of these excuses by avoiding the possibility of any extended relationships with the stranger. He is using alcohol to alleviate further expectations and responsibilities in exchanging information. These are workable compromises if the usage is moderate, and are common tuning techniques for millions of individuals. Ralph gives the impression that he will walk out of the bar feeling better than when he walked in.

Escape Techniques That Increase Tension

Most excuse clauses are productive on a temporary basis if not exclusively used in attempt to escape responsibility totally. Some escape techniques may prolong the dissynchrony within the individual by perpetuating an already unvalidatable self concept. The anxious or tense person is already experiencing the stress of an unrealistic self-concept and his frantic attempts to escape incorporating unwanted data in his self-concept may leave him even more vulnerable to continued threats by compromising his ability to exchange information with others. He is forced to limit his data-exchange system to those persons who will not threaten him or who will give him help on a superficial level. This isolation may further impoverish his poor self-esteem.

The following vignette is given as an illustration of the threatened self-concept of a particular individual and his unsuccessful efforts to lower tension. This situation is analogous to the interaction in the bar. Again, the advantage to the speaker is that of the transiency of the situation, although it is less safe than the stranger in the bar because the two individuals do know each other on a much more intimate basis. The speaker might feel a little less inhibited, owing to his friend's profession and the improbability of prolonged intimacy.

Rusty! Hey, Russ! Hell, doggone, son of a gun it is you! How the hell have you been, Russ? . . . Jesus, I thought it was you but you know I almost walked right past. You haven't changed a bit, a few gray hairs, but what the hell? . . . Say, you're a psychiatrist now, huh? You even look like a psychiatrist. Just kidding. . . . Have time for a cup of coffee or a drink? My plane leaves in half an hour. . . . No kidding, are you going to D.C. too? Son of a—. Great, that gives us a couple of hours to chew the rag. How long has it been? . . . At least that. Let's see—we graduated in '57 and we finished our internship in July '58 and we met at that convention when we were house officers. It's been at least twelve years. It doesn't seem that long. . . . Well, sometimes it seems like an eternity. . . . I bumped into Pete Legget a year or so ago and he told me you were practicing in Dallas. I'm sorry to hear about your wife. . . . I never met her. Pete said she was really a sweet kid. It was leukemia, wasn't it? . . . Bad break. . . . Oh, you're married again? Great. . . . That's just great. A boy and a girl. You can't beat that combination. . . . Just one, a boy. You remember, he was born when we were sophomores in medical school. . . . Let's see, he's about seventeen now. He's a big kid; at least he was the last time I saw him a few months ago. . . . No, Lois and I split up a few years back. . . . Well, it was one of those things. I guess we just weren't compatible, whatever the hell that means. . . . No, that's a cop-out. The fact is I blew the relationship. You know how it is when you're the dashing young house officer. All the nurses and nursing students imply you're a good catch and pretty soon you begin to believe it yourself and tease a few along just for the ride. A lot of guys are able to keep things on a superficial level, but I began to think I'd been cheated out of really exploring the field. . . . Say, that's our plane. Maybe we can get a seat together if it's okay with you. . . . Great. . . . Yeah, I like these with exits even though I bet they put the emergency doors in solely for psychological reasons. . . . Hell, you know this bird stalls at 250 miles an hour—. . . . When we stop, we either use the regular exit or somebody outside uses a can opener. . . . Like I was saying back there in the terminal, I guess I blew it. Say, you don't mind me talking about it, do you? You always were a good listener, and, besides, you're in psychiatry . . . . Lois always liked you. You remember you used to come over so we could study anatomy and physiology and Lois would spend half the damn evening telling you what Billy did or bitching about not having any money or time together. I guess we were in more trouble even then than we thought. . . . I know it didn't show, but she was starting to get jealous even then. She really was overly possessive. . . . Well, she came from a well-to-do family you know, and in many ways she was a spoiled brat. She never did break loose from her mother. That didn't become evident until her father died. He was really a nice guy. He owned a lot of those buildings across from main campus. Dropped dead on the golf course. Coronary, I guess. Anyway, Lois was the only child and it more or less threw her and her mother together. . . . Let's see, we were interning at the time and I had a pretty heavy call schedule. I almost lived in the hospital and Lois and her mother almost lived at the Country Club. I guess that's when she really began to get jealous of me. Looking back, I blame her mother for a lot of it. Her mother always drank pretty heavy but

when the old man died she began to border on being a lush.
Lois was drinking then, too. I could always tell when she was
drinking too much. She would call me at the hospital and ask
how the nurses were. I was working damned hard those days
bucking for rank, you know. Lois used to try to convince me
that she inherited enough money and that I was a fool for
busting my ass at the hospital, but, hell, I didn't want to feel like
a gigolo. Maybe I was working too hard. I don't know what it
was but I had a little trouble with impotency that year and she
used to fly into a rage and accuse me of stepping out on her.
I'm sure that damned mother of hers didn't help. She was
probably horny after her husband died and tried to live
vicariously through Lois. I don't know. That's what the marriage
counselor we went to a year or so later said. Sounds good,
whatever it means. Anyway, she began to start teasing me. She
and her mother would talk about the life guard at the country
club and make innuendos about affairs and that sort of crap. I'm
sure that Lois was really jealous of me and trying to make me
jealous but, if anything, it only made me angry and I got more
impotent. But at a time like that, you can't let a woman get the
upper hand, or Christ, she'll lead you around by the nose the
rest of your life. So I told her if she wanted to screw around
that it was her nickel but not to come whining around to me if
she got herself knocked up. I think that hurt her but she's
almost as stubborn as I am so she and her mother started
staying out evenings. At least she said she was with her mother.
Hell, what difference does it make? If she was that jealous
maybe it's a good thing we broke up. Anyway, I began hearing
rumors. Maybe you heard some of them. That internship year
was a hell of a year for me. We didn't see each other as much
that year, did we? . . . You were always on different services
from me somehow. Then you went to Colorado the next year in
psychiatry and I stayed on in surgery. The latter part of our
internship year I met a girl named Joan and we got pretty close.
You probably won't believe it but it was a platonic thing. She
was a few years older than me and the psychiatrist I was going
to then for my damned impotence made a big deal about an
Oedipal complex. However, Lois really hit the ceiling when I told
her about Joan. She was so jealous of me you wouldn't believe
it. I told her I wasn't upset about the rumors that were going on
about her and some of the house staff. You know, she actually
laughed when I told her about Joan, but I know she was
laughing to cover up her tremendous jealousy. God, talk about
the green-eyed monster, she had it. We more or less went our
own ways after that. I talked her into seeing a marriage
counselor with me because I wanted to make sure I didn't hurt
her but she was already too hurt. She laughted about the
sessions. That was her way of denying the pain. My psychiatrist
agreed with me on that point. Billy's had a little problem with
drugs but I'm sure he'll straighten up. Got good breeding! He'll

be a chip off the old block, you wait. What do you know, he's starting his descent into Washington. There's the "No Smoking" sign. Say, Russ, could I ask you something personal? . . . I mean, if you'd rather not answer, don't. . . . Well, I've been curious. Did you ever sleep with Lois? . . . Well, don't get defensive. If you did, you did. Who the hell cares, anyway? Even if you did, you'd probably never tell anyone to protect Lois. . . . Well, don't get uptight; I believe you. It's not like it's a big issue. Just a matter of curiosity. . . . No, I never heard it implied that you did, or if I did, I've forgotten it. Anyway, maybe it was all rumors. You don't know of any situation where she was actually shacking up with any of the guys, do you? . . . I didn't think you would tell me. You're too nice a guy to say, anyway. At one time I used to think you were a smug son-of-a-bitch but now I realize you were only trying to keep from hurting my feelings. . . . Don't give me that. You know what I mean. . . . Okay, if you insist on playing it that way. I don't care if you're still screwing her, you hear me? There isn't a damn thing that bitch can do to make me jealous. Let her eat her heart out, I don't give a damn. I wouldn't take her back if she crawled back on her hands and knees. . . . Oh, I'm sorry. I guess I am getting a little loud. Sorry, stewardess. How long are you going to be in Washington? . . . Yeah, me too. Sorry we don't have time for a drink or something. Good to see you again. And say, if you're ever through Pittsburgh again, give me a call. Okay? . . . See ya!

It is apparent in this vignette that the speaker is involved in a crisis situation. He is having some difficulty in adjusting his self-concept as required by the events in his life. He is almost desperately trying to escape his responsibility for the dissynchrony in his self system. His inability to make the needed shifts in his self-concept not only interrupted his life style but posed a severe threat to one of the roles composing his self system, that is, the role of a sexually adequate male. He attempts to escape incorporating information implying his inadequacy as a sexual partner by focusing on his wife's jealousy and blaming his mother-in-law for marital discord.

His persistent insecurity and its concomitant anxiety is evident in the emotionally charged questions at the end of the conversation. His frantic attempt to obtain information that will help him explain the bewildering circumstances without reorganizing his self-concept almost reaches paranoid level when he implies that his friend may have participated in the break-up of his marriage or may be withholding vital information concerning the event. Although a great deal of information was exchanged in this example of an effort at self-tuning, we may postulate that both participants left the interchange with a higher level of anxiety.

In this example, unlike the previous one, the speaker attempts to make his listener at least partially responsible for his misery. He communicates that he expects help in the solution of his problem. This subtle attempt at controlling how the relationship is to be defined may have alienated the person with whom he was trying to exchange the information.

Almost all persons, at some time in their life spans, must adjust to the loss of a significant other, whether that loss occurs through death or through the inability of the individuals to synchronize their behavioral paradigms. Most of these adjustments are made without the intervention of outside professional help, although it is more difficult without the help of others in the information-exchange system.

Use of Property Some individuals use property as a mode of making their self-concepts more secure. The relationship between the individual self system, other self systems, and concrete and abstract objects that are owned is complex. "Ownership" is an interaction in which an individual defines objects and relationships as property, for example, my spouse, my friend, my house, and my idea. This gives the illusion that the individual is controlling the relationship. On closer scrutiny, we can appreciate that these properties further delineate and define the boundaries of the individual's self system and, therefore, exert a reciprocal type of control. The real or threatened loss of property endangers the individual's self-esteem, causing him to be at the mercy of that property.

A threat to property may result in anxiety because the property is now seen by the individual as a part of his self-concept. This anxiety may cause the individual to focus more on property as a technique of control and prediction of future self-referencing information. Frantic acquisition of property, whether the property be scientific data or financial affluence, rigidifies the self-boundaries, increasing the potential for threatened loss. For example, a scientist may become distraught when someone takes credit for his ideas and the businessman may become despondent when his capital is devalued. An individual whose self system includes other family members as property may become extremely anxious when his spouse becomes interested in another relationship or the children leave home.

The adaptation of a life style of acquiring property is not necessarily dysfunctional, however, and may be an acceptable mode of living for some people.

Other Common Adjustment Techniques   Some common techniques used by individuals as tuning mechanisms besides the use of alcohol or other drugs and the acquisition of property include among others, devotion to a cause, service to others, work, sex, education, recreation, and various forms of religion. All of these adjustment techniques may help the individual self system to exist with some illusion of autonomy and to gratify the need for synchrony within a particular social system. Such tuning mechanisms are helpful in allaying dissynchrony and allowing the individual to live through stressful situations with a minimum of discomfort. When the self system is severely or continuously stressed, self-tuning techniques may take the form of self-perpetuating dissynchrony.

Reference   1. Deikman, A. *Personal freedom: On finding your way to the real world*. New York: Viking, 1976, P. 4.

Suggested Readings   Arieti, S. (Ed.), *American handbook of psychiatry*, Vols. I, II, and III. New York: Basic Books, 1974.

Benton, A. Psychological tests for brain damage. In A. Freedman, H. Kaplan, and B. Sadock (Eds.), *Comprehensive textbook of psychiatry/II*, Vol. I. Baltimore: Williams and Wilkins, 1975.

Cooley, C. The social self. In T. Parsons, E. Shils, K. Naegele, and J. Pitts (Eds.), *Theories of society: foundations of modern sociological theory*, Vol. II. New York: Free Press, 1961.

Hine, F. *Introduction to psychodynamics: a conflict-adaptational approach*. Durham, North Carolina: Duke University Press, 1971.

Horney, K. *The neurotic personality of our time*. New York: W. W. Norton, 1937.

Kolb, L. *Modern clinical psychiatry*. Philadelphia, Pennsylvania: W. B. Saunders, 1973.

Lederer, W., and Jackson, D. *The mirages of marriage*. New York: W. W. Norton, 1968.

Masters, W., and Johnson, V. *Human sexual inadequacy*. Boston: Little, Brown, 1970.

Reich, W. *Character analysis*. New York: The Noonday Press, Farrar, Straws and Cudahy, 1962.

Suggested Questions

1. Give a definition of human behavior.
2. Give three disadvantages which use of the self-referencing apparatus has allowed man.
3. Give a definition of life style.
4. Do you think that it is possible for two people to be exactly alike? Why or why not?
5. Give two factors that may result in individuals claiming they are never under stress or have no problems.
6. When may crises in our lives occur? Give examples.
7. Discuss the utilization of people by people. Give an example.
8. Define excuse clauses.
9. State the primary function of an excuse clause.
10. Give your own example of an escape technique that might increase tension.
11. Discuss the integration of property into one's self-concept.
12. Name several other common adjustment techniques used by individuals as tuning mechanisms besides the use of alcohol and other drugs and the acquisition of property.

9 Dissynchronous Behavior

> . . . human behavior is the expression of a dynamic interrelationship between the individual and his environment at a particular point in time and space . . . mental health and the various deviations therefrom are but expressions of varying quantitative aspects of this relationship which at certain crucial levels results in quantitative changes.
>
> Judd Marmor and Eugene Pumpian-Mindlin, 1969 (4)

Response to Injury   As we have noted in previous chapters, the self system develops slowly over a period of time, adopting certain life styles that give it a sense of autonomy. The evolving self system is continually making adjustments to life situations in order to maintain a state of equilibrium. To state this thought in yet another way, to remain in synchrony or harmony with the environment, each individual makes fine-tuning adjustments as the need arises.

Most of us have minimal difficulty staying in synchrony, and find ourselves out of harmony only occasionally. All of us are susceptible to the stresses and strains of everyday living and all of us exhibit behaviors at times which might be termed "unusual," "strange," or "weird." These terms denote behaviors that differentiate us from each other and that may depart slightly from what is commonly described as "normal." These behaviors may or may not be associated with discomfort.

When the information that emanates from a self system indicates prolonged discomfort in the individual and/or produces discomfort in others, it may be termed *dissynchronous.* For some, dissynchrony is of such magnitude that it results in patterns of behavior that have been termed *mental illness.* Mental illness is an abstraction denoting a condition in which the individual is so out of tune with his environment that he may need professional help in order to return to a state of equilibrium.

Persons experience uneasiness or anxiety when the analogic and digital readout of their information coding processes, that is, their nonverbal and verbal communication patterns, are out of synchrony with those about them. This dissynchrony may lead to confusion in the definition of relationships and a lack of predictability in the information-exchange system.

Dissynchronous behavior can be divided into two major categories: (*a*) those behaviors resulting from injury to the physiologic coding equipment (for example, brain damage) and (*b*) those behaviors resulting from disruption of any of the subsystems of data organization that contribute to the data bank we have termed the self system (for example, loss of employment or flunking out of school).

Dissynchronous behaviors can be viewed simultaneously as unsuccessful tuning techniques and as signals emanating from a self system that has been injured or is under threat of injury. Pathophysiology can be defined as a dynamic interaction of tissues and injurious circumstances. Using this conceptual framework, tuberculosis is not the invasion of the human organism by the tubercle bacillus but the dynamic interaction of these two living systems, which only occasionally produces an injury and reaction to injury sufficient to produce the symptoms and signs that we refer to as a *disease process* (1). This mode of conceptualization allows the student more flexibility than the concrete delineation of tuberculosis or other diseases as distinct and well-defined entities.

Injury to the physiologic coding equipment usually causes injury to the self system. For example, the onset of any disease and its subsequent course will produce changes in self-concept of either minor or major consequence, depending on the severity of the disease. Cancer would probably produce major changes in self-concept (for example, "I am a dying person"), whereas a bad cold might produce only minor changes (for example, "I am too sick to care what I look like"), and those only for the duration of the disease process. Injury to the self system *may* produce physiologic disturbances in some individuals. For example, the student who flunks out of school and thus begins to view himself as a failure may develop ulcers or headaches or any number of physiological symptoms. Injury to the physiologic coding equipment alters the self system just as injury to the self system alters the physiologic coding equipment.

Losses or threatened losses of key sources of data, whether these data come from inside or outside the organism, may cause radical shifts in the self system. Dissynchronous behaviors, then, are a response to real or threatened injury to the self. The injury and the response are types of coded information.

Continual Exchange of Data

In addressing dissynchronous behavior as coded information, we will focus mainly on the codes exchanged through interpersonal communications. However, we would like to call attention to our original thesis that all of the information coding systems, ranging from complex social interactions to equally complex inter- and intracellular activity, are continually exchanging data. The data move from one mode of coding to another, with continuous feedback loops.

All human behavior must be viewed as a physiologic process. Dissynchronous behavior, like any other behavior, results in and/or from shifts in the physiologic coding systems. The introduction of chemical agents into the coding apparatus results in information that alters behavior. Some of the most exciting scientific advances are coming from studies of the biochemical coding systems that influence the behavioral readout. Neural transmitting substances, which play a prominent role in the information coding continuum, have been the focus of recent attention.

Pharmacologic agents, for example, the MAO inhibitors, tricyclic antidepressants, phenothiazines, butyrophenones, and lithium carbonate provide new instruments for altering the biochemical coding systems and realigning the information flow to ameliorate dissynchronous behavior. Other chemicals, such as the hallucinogens, are now available for disrupting standard behavioral patterns and producing dissynchronous behavior.

All these reagents may be considered as information. How this information interacts with the data-processing systems within the individual is one of the most exciting questions confronting students of behavior.

Analog to Digital Impasse

We postulated in Chapter 3 that the information-processing systems in the human can be conceptualized as two major systems, the analog system and the digital system. These systems are synchronized in the analog-to-digital ratio at any given time, depending on the individual's state of arousal. If the information processed by each of the two systems is not synchronized, an impasse may result.

An analog-to-digital impasse may begin to "heat up" the data-processing system, resulting in cybernetic dissynchrony, that is, symptoms such as anxiety or depression. This is a signal to the organism to exert greater effort in synchronizing these two systems. This signal increases the state of arousal and may increase efficiency to a point. If the arousal passes the point of maximal efficiency, there is a shift in the analog-to-digital ratio toward the analog, decreasing the efficiency and resulting in a fight–flight paradigm of retreat from, or attack on, stimuli that cannot be programmed.

When any animal, including man, becomes anxious, tense, or fearful, it prepares itself either to run away or to attack. The fight–flight pattern is often a useful program for handling stressful situations when it is a transient state (more or less like a fire drill), and if the individual settles down when his perceptual inputs and coding equipment register that it is no longer necessary to run or to fight.

To illustrate, a student facing an examination of major consequence might feel a slight increase in anxiety level, signaling a need to think about the subject matter and study in time for the test. If the anxiety increases to the point where the student cannot rest, eat, or concentrate on studying, the shift toward the analog has passed the point of maximum efficiency and he begins to "spin his wheels," unable to synchronize his analog and digital coding systems so that he can expend the energy in studying. Energy is being expended but it is being spent in pacing the floor, worrying, and running from the situation.

In extreme cases of anxiety, the use of pharmacologic agents (for example, sedatives or tranquilizers) may decrease the state of arousal resulting in a more productive analog-to-digital ratio.

If the energy expended in coping efforts has resulted in a decreased state of arousal and a shift toward the analog, other medications (for example, antidepressants) may be useful in energizing the system and reestablishing a functional analog-to-digital ratio. For example, the student whose efforts to cope with an examination result in immobilization may exhibit symptoms of depression. The student may sit and stare into space, will not talk, and experiences changes in sleep patterns. This shift toward the analog is also unproductive.

It is rather common for persons experiencing symptoms resulting from an analog-to-digital impasse to resort to chemical agents for assistance. The danger in using chemical agents resides in the possibility that escape from the painful anxiety necessary for learning may result in a phobia (fear) about anxiety so that when the individual is again confronted by a similar impasse he may attempt to avoid it by medication rather than learning to negotiate or integrate the data (stimuli) in an harmonic analog and digital paradigm.

Students will often appear in college and university health services around exam time asking for some kind of medication to alleviate their anxiety. If they do receive a chemical agent that helps, they may continue to rely on this agent every time they face an examination rather than submit themselves to the anxiety, which is a natural state for almost all students at that particular time. It is easier, then, to begin to resort to medication in order to alleviate anxiety at other times as when giving a talk or anticipating new situations (for example, a blind date). This dependency is a result of the growing phobia (fear) about anxiety that the student is experiencing.

As has been previously stated, symptoms arise when the analog and digital processing of data in a social system is not synchronized. It must be emphasized that digital data processing is heavily dependent on group validation. When the individual's digital operation is not synchronized with the group in which he lives, the disharmony results in anxiety and fight–flight patterns. Disruption of a group's information-processing activity can arise from dissynchrony between the analog and digital readouts of one or more of the members. This is often seen in family communication problems, when the nonverbal communication arising from the analog of individual group members does not match the digital or linguistic symbols they send out.

Dependency on Group Interaction

Being human depends on group interaction and how well we have learned the roles and counterroles that help us to be accepted in the groups in which we live. Our communication system is the tool that we use to validate our roles in a social or group structure. The human has evolved into a rather gregarious creature and shows signs and symptoms of anxiety or fear when isolated from a group. All humans are products of groups and are continually relating to a group, whether it is the present group, or a group of persons stored in memory banks—parents, teachers, peers, and significant others. Individuals need to be able to predict how people are going to relate to them or they become somewhat anxious and tense.

If tension reaches a sufficient level they enter the fight–flight pattern. Usually, the human animal runs and fights abstractly. He either makes peace or convinces other people that he is correct. But those few individuals who are never quite able to reach a homeostatic or stabilized situation may maintain a set of being ready to fight or flee. This puts a great deal of stress on many systems within the individual organism, so that, sooner or later, there are signs of tissue and behavioral reactions called symptoms. Continual stress may produce gastrointestinal symptoms associated with ulceration of the duodenum or stomach or increased motility of the bowel as in mucous colitis. There may be spasms of the smooth muscles in the respiratory system called asthma, vascular involvement leading to high blood pressure, and muscle tension resulting in back pain, joint pain and other symptoms of distress. This type of tissue reaction on continued stress has been called a *psychophysiologic phenomenon* or psychophysiologic disease.

Attempts to Avoid Expectations

Under stress, the anxious individual attempts to avoid the pressure of expectations, including those he has incorporated in his own self system and those of other self systems which require responsible behavior. One of the most common escape techniques is the emission of behavior that communicates a total dependency on others. This type of behavior resembles that of a young child. When it occurs in an adult it has been termed *regression*.

A similar, but more disturbing pattern of behavior that avoids expectations and responsibilities is the disjointed nonlogical communication seen in the panicked individual. If significant others show concern, this attention may decrease his anxiety and make him feel more secure so that he can learn more efficiently. In some cases, this concern in itself may be a type of attention that reinforces nonresponsible behavior. Validation of this pattern over a period of time may allow the individual to incorporate this behavioral readout into his self system, with diminished capacity for defining relationships other than those in which he is responsible. This dependent state increases the individual's vulnerability, in that other individuals in his society may resent the increased expectations on their self systems to care for this parasitic individual.

If the resentment toward a symptomatic individual takes the form of expressed hostility or avoidance, the individual may feel rejected and more tense and anxious, catalyzing the emission of more irresponsible behavior. Patterns of behavior emanated in this state of dependency range from the childlike theatrical communications that are termed *hysterical* or *dissociative* to the autistic, loosely associated, ambivalent behavior termed *schizophrenic*, with its inappropriate affective tone. The cause of irresponsible behaviors by certain individuals under stress is at present a matter of speculation. Many theories give poorly learned interpersonal skills as a causal factor, whereas other theories imply a genetic defect and/or a metabolic derangement. These theories do not preclude the possibility of multiple overlapping causal factors.

So long as the information-exchange system is fairly stable and the role–counterrole constellations are predictable, the individual self system is able to participate with minimal adjustments. Where there are major or untimely shifts in the exchange system brought about by increasing or decreasing membership in the exchange or by changes in a participant's data-programming apparatus (for example, alteration of the central nervous system), all the participants are driven by their information hunger to reorganize relationships that have been disrupted by unanticipated information. The frustrated individual frantically attempts to realign his self system with the information available, so that previously programmed information may allow predictable anticipation of future data. If his attempts are continually thwarted, this behavior may become increasingly dissynchronous, being unpredictable both to himself and to others. He is then out of synchrony with the group.

Classification of Behavioral Patterns

In studying human behavior, we learn to classify those patterns of behavior that are characteristic of individuals who are out of tune or in disharmony with the information-exchange system of their social environment. Emil Kraepelin's work in cataloging various patterns of behavior emanating from dissynchronous individuals gives the illusion that these patterns represent discrete entities (2, p. 408; 3).

Thomas Szaz in his book *The Myth of Mental Illness* decrys the rigid disease model as a way of viewing behavior (5). However, if we abdicate the concept of illness, we must not abdicate the idea that dissynchronous behaviors resulting from injuries to self-concept can cause as much or more pain and suffering in the individual and his family and community as any purely physiological disturbance.

We believe that all illness can be productively viewed as a response to injury. One advantage of using the "response to injury" model is that it allows us to maintain the flexibility to understand that the same type of injury may evoke different behaviors in different individuals or that different injuries may evoke patterns of behavior that are indistinguishable in a given individual or different individuals.

In addressing man's physiological and emotional reactions to injury, we may find categorization helpful in comprehending and communicating rapidly about various patterns of behavior, so long as we remain aware that these classifications are working constructs, "as if" propositions, and not absolutes or rigidly defined entities.

Individuals who are desperately trying to synchronize their self systems with the information emanating from their memory banks and from their environments may emit a wide range of behaviors, including hyperalert searching activity, which we might term *anxiety;* frustrated withdrawal, which we might term *depression;* or the more chaotic and fragmented patterns of communication which we call *psychotic.*

In the latter, the individual's communication techniques may be so distorted by his fight–flight pattern of attempting to synchronize himself that we say that he no longer "tests reality." Here again there is a tendency to assume that reality is an entity rather than an "as if" working construct that a given social unit agrees upon as guidelines in the information-exchange system. An individual who developed a new reality system that programmed information more efficiently than the one of his culture might be termed psychotic if he were unable to synchronize this new method with that of his social system.

For example, a student who continually talked in such abstract and incomprehensible terms that he alienated his peer group might be termed "crazy" because he refuses to make his views known in such a way as to be understood. Although he might be considered a genius in some circles, he might be seen as psychotic by those who cannot follow him. As the student becomes more alienated from his peer group, he may exhibit other behaviors that seem strange. In his attempts to "belong," he may only succeed in appearing more strange.

Genius is often compared to insanity. Although this comparison has merit, one would expect that the individual with a more efficient data-processing system and hence better facilities for prediction would be less anxious or show fewer signs of disorganization. This is not usually the case of the individuals termed psychotic. There is good evidence that those persons exhibiting behaviors that have been called psychotic have organizational deficits, perhaps stemming from the genetic program of their central nervous system, which makes it difficult for them to program all the contingencies existing in the information-exchange system. Whether this deficit disrupts perception, the analogic coding of data, or the analog-to-digital conversion of data necessary for language is at present uncertain. The attempts of an individual exhibiting psychotic behavior to tune himself with the social system are further compromised by spiraling anxiety, which decreases his ability to exchange information with others. In this situation, the coping techniques that the individual uses to tune himself may become a detriment to synchronization.

Panic shifts the analog-to-digital ratio of data programming toward the analog side, making linear logic and the cause-and-effect paradigm usually necessary for communication difficult. The individual now groping wildly to arrange his information into a predictable sequence may select cause-and-effect relationships that cannot be validated by the members in his society.

To illustrate, the person who is in a state of panic and is exhibiting dissynchronous behavior may begin to believe that the CIA is the cause of his problems and will state that, "They are out to get me." Or he will pick some other group of persons or some single person as causing his discomfort. He seems unable to think in a logical manner or to use any sequential reasoning to explain his acute distress.

These distorted cause-and-effect sequences have been termed *paranoia,* a process that further alienates the individual from a synchronized data base.

In summary, when we address clinical syndromes, that is, dysfunctional behavioral patterns, we must take into account three major factors:

1. How the data are organized.
2. The state of arousal and emotional tone associated with the data organized.
3. The effect the readout of this data organization has on other persons.

Dissynchronous data organization occurs when the central nervous system is defective, damaged, or given stimuli that it has difficulty in organizing, that is, subjected to stress.

If the data organization is so dissynchronous that others are unable to understand the behavioral readout, the individual may be called psychotic. Psychotic behavioral patterns have been classified into several subgroups including schizophrenia, mania, depression, and organic brain syndromes. Severe disorganization or loose association of information with socially inappropriate emotional tone has been termed *schizophrenic.* An elevated state of arousal associated with data in such a way as to imply that the individual is extremely important may reach sufficient state of grandiosity to be termed *mania.* The converse, that is, decreased emotional tone and data organization indicating severe self-deprecation and despondency is called *psychotic depression.* Disruption of the data organization resulting in memory loss and inability to predict subsequent data, that is, impaired judgment, may stem from any acute or chronic brain injury and is termed an *organic brain syndrome.*

Regardless of the category, the term psychosis implies a behavioral pattern in which the individual is not testing or experiencing "reality" in the manner that others of the same age, sex, and culture do. All other emotional disturbances of lesser degree have as a common factor a system of information exchange that is dissynchronous with that of significant others.

We must be careful in describing behavioral patterns lest we establish these descriptions or diagnoses as entities, that is, closed systems. The closed systems approach to human behavior has had a distorting effect on the study of and response to persons suffering the discomfort of dissynchronous behavior.

Inability to Accept Help

Individuals who are suffering from an untuned self system and its resulting dissynchronized data-processing systems are often subjected to platitudes from well-meaning bystanders. These include such phrases as "Get hold of yourself," "You are trying to be difficult," or "You should face reality." While these abortive therapeutic attempts may seem logical to the individual who is in tune with society, they indicate that the observer still expects the individual whom he is addressing to have a well-delineated and concretized self system somewhere hidden in the "back of his mind," which can emerge on command and take charge of the situation.

These expectations result from failure to comprehend that the self system is a crucial part of the data-programming organization and faulty organization of information and an inept self system are often one and the same. In the early stages of self-discord, the individual may tune himself by sharing information with others. However, in the late stages of this spiral of disorganized information programming, the individual self system may be in such disarray that even the need for synchronization is unprogrammable. In the latter case, the responsibility for synchronizing the individual's behavior now rests on significant others.

Effects of Institutionalization

In order to establish a homeostatic relationship between the fragmented self system and information from the outside, it may be advisable to relieve the individual of the stress of expectations and to decrease the panic by pharmacologic agents to a level where the analog-to-digital ratio allows a logical sequence for "reality testing." Prior to the advent of pharmacologic agents, psychotic individuals were removed from society and placed in institutions with other psychotic individuals. Although this may have, in some instances, relieved the expectations, the information obtained from other psychotic individuals was so chaotic in nature that realignment of the self systems of those involved was markedly compromised. Tragically, in some instances, rather than a relief of expectations, the individuals were subjected to institutional expectations, at least covertly. The expectations of the institutions became again a self-fulfilling prophecy, that is, "Since you are crazy we expect you to act crazy." Uncrazy behavior was often seen as being unpredictable and somewhat threatening to the institution keepers.

Unpredictable and crazy behaviors then became the social norm of institutions erected by a social system to care for shattered self systems. Institutionalized persons who have been termed psychotic develop, perhaps inadvertently, communication patterns that may control relationships. They seem to be aware of the responses that will draw significant others closer to them and they seem aware of the responses that will have the effect of giving them distance. It is not unusual to hear personnel in institutions argue the question of whether or not certain persons diagnosed as psychotic are not perhaps more aware of the effects of their communication techniques than they admit. This can perhaps be illustrated by the following vignette in which it appears that the patient is quite aware of what he is saying.

What are you anyway? A social worker, psychologist, psychiatrist, what? . . . Oh, a social worker. You know, some of my best friends are social workers. Maybe even God's a social worker. . . . I'm sorry. I just, I don't know, well, I've just seen so many people come and go. Maybe I'm not even really a people. As a matter of fact, I think this is an unpeople place. This is where they put unpeople and they call some of the unpeople patients and some of the unpeople staff. Maybe there's a place where people go backstage and change their costumes. . . . Say, I mean seriously, are you one of us in disguise or are you a spy for one of them? . . . Oh, that omnipotent "they" out there that expects us to do something. I mean, it's as though we're in a cage and they throw us peanuts. . . . I suppose it does sound like crazy talk to you. Well, that's because I am, shall we say, a bit—deranged? At least that's what they have intimated for the past several years. Either that or there has been a tremendous injustice done to me, because I now believe they are correct in their assumption that I am crazy. I am not certain that they are not crazy also, but they have the keys and I do not. Let's see, you asked me why I'm here. Perhaps the all-wise God and His wife, Mother Nature, built me for this place. Would you believe perhaps I was made for the state hospital. . . . Oh, my hands? Well, I used to think it was the cosmic rays that made them red like that, but Dr. Whatshisname, Zhivago or something, has convinced me that I wash them too much. And I do. I wash the hell out of them all the time. I mean, I don't know, they feel dirty. I mean, like they've got germs crawling on them. Everything seems dirty, I mean, like you know everything smells like sex or feces. You smell it in here? I mean, it's all over everything. . . . No, I'm not putting you on. I mean, I'm not saying you could smell it if you wanted to or that I could stop smelling it if I wanted to, I'm just calling it like it is. . . . Well, it's kinda difficult to talk about it, I mean, since you're a woman and all, but I think it really is a part of my problem. I think I got a problem because I never did have genuine sexual intercourse

with anyone except myself. I can't get it off my mind, but I never
did. I have had sexual contact with women but never true
intercourse. I masturbate a great deal, both physically and
mentally, if you know what I mean? Do you think I'll go blind?
. . . You don't, huh? Well, I don't really either. I don't see any
change in my eyesight and I've been doing it for many years,
but maybe it has to reach critical mass or something and, then,
zang! All of a sudden the lights go out and there I am, holding
my penis in my hand. . . . No, I don't really believe it, but you
know, you get a sense of humor after a while. I used to take this
stuff awfully serious, but you see so damn many doctors come
and go and social workers and things. I don't know. I guess I
could sit around and blow bubbles. I'm all mixed up. There's no
shit about that. Excuse my language, please, but it has
deteriorated along with everything else. Sometimes it's like I
almost understand everything. . . . The ironic part is that when
I feel like I understand, it scares the whaley out of me. That's
the most frightening time of all, when I think I understand. Isn't
that a Goddamned pity? The great force that shaped the cosmos
chose to enlighten only one of his earthly creatures and that
little son-of-a-bitch has been canned in a state hospital. . . .
Oh, really, I knew better than that. I was just putting you on. I
really was putting you on that time. . . . I mean, no, I'm sorry, I
didn't aim to, you know, be off base or anything like that. . . .
No, I haven't been here the whole time. I mean, they let me go
back to mommie and the farm several times. They even let me
go to my father's funeral. The poor devil hanged himself. As a
matter of fact, I've been discharged three or four times, but I
always come creeping back. I get panicky, you know? You
probably won't believe this, but I'm pretty uptight right now. I
mean, I can feel my armpits sweating. . . . Oh, I know you're
not going to hurt me. I know that. I know people love me and
want me and that sort of thing, but there's a force, excuse my
physics but I've read a lot of science fiction since I've been here
and this force is working against my security and I can't tell
whether it's inside me or outside me, but I have learned that if I
say it's outside of me they increase my Stelazine or Thorazine or
Mellaril or whatever damn drug I happen to be on, so let's say
that the force is inside me and it keeps me from believing what I
know. Does that make any sense, I mean, believing what I
know? Okay, okay. . . . You want to go all the way back to the
beginning? God, I've been over it so many times. I mean, no
offense meant. I can't even remember myself. I've even read
some psychiatric books and I can't separate now what is my
dynamics from what is their dynamics. I even read Noyes and
Kolb. My doctor, Zhivago I call him, lent it to me. . . . Oh, I call
him that because he can't speak English. He's really not a bad
sort really. I mean, if you give him a lot of time to think. Anyway
in Noyes and Kolb, which they tell me is their Bible, I am a
classic schizophrenic and Dr. Noyes and Dr. Kolb, whoever they

are, can sure spot one. You know, the lonely child that tried to
please and all that. You know, I think that's the key, lonely. I've
always been lonely, really. If I could have had one friend, if I
could have had just one friend, I don't think I would be
here. . . . I tried, yes, I've tried very hard to have friends. I was
near the top of my class all the way through high school. I even
went out for the basketball team, but I don't know, it always
came out badly. You know, when I went out on a date, it
seemed like I wasn't really with it. On the basketball court or at
parties I felt everybody was looking at me and I froze up and the
older I got, the more hell it became. You know, I still have
nightmares, I mean, still nightmares about the examinations and
the dates and crap like that. Boy, I had a doozey last night. I
dreamed I was at a trading post or something like that and there
was this big, black woman and she was naked with her vagina
showing. I mean, it looked like it was leather, and she suggested
since we were both royalty that we have intercourse, only when
I pulled out my penis it had a fingernail on top of it and when I
put it in her vagina, it went soft because it kept bumping
against rice and pieces of food in there. Isn't that a hell of a
dream? But at any rate, in the middle of this frightening
phenomena, it seemed like we were in church and John
Kennedy was there and I was singing and it was echoing. You
know, you could hear it like "Student Prince." Now, if that isn't
a schizophrenic dream, you won't ever hear one, right? What do
you think, doc? I mean, mam'm, or whatever you're called.
Soch. How about that, Soch? Well, I woke up sweating and sick
and everytime I get scared I smell it, like I now smell sex in
here. I think about things like that and then it makes me feel
even more scared and sick. I know it's all pathological, but I
can't stop thinking about it. You know what I really think? I
think I'm a queer. I've been afraid for a long time that I was a
queer. . . . No, I never had intercourse with a male. I never had
true intercourse with anyone except myself. I am always afraid,
though, that someday I'm going to grab somebody and kiss him
on the face or neck or rip open his fly or something like that. I
can't control myself. . . . No, we can talk about my mother
later. I've talked about my mother until I'm tired of talking about
my mother. If she's schizophrenogenic, I can't help being
schizophrenic, and all that. I mean, she couldn't help it any
more than I can help it and I'm sick of it. If we talk about my
wife you'll say she was castrating but I won't believe it because I
don't think there was ever anything there to castrate. I'm talking
abstractly, of course. Besides, she's married again. You know
what I really think did it? You know, I think the turning point in
my life was one time when I and these other two kids were
playing. I mean, we were playing down in an old barn on the
farm next to where we lived and there was this horse, I mean,
there was this old mare, and the other two kids were bigger
than me and they tied this old mare by her head. She was very

gentle and all, so she didn't really mind, and then the biggest boy got a crate and he stuck his penis in her. She seemed to like it because she held her tail up and then the other guy, the other kid, did it and then they asked me to do it and I couldn't do it and I wanted to run. I was afraid to even look at my penis, but I couldn't keep from looking at theirs and I thought about penises a lot and that's why I think I'm a queer because every now and then I see their penises, I mean, in my mind I can see their penises going in and out of that black vagina, that big horse, I mean, with her holding her tail up and all. And it excites me, but it makes me sick. I sometimes think about it when I masturbate. Anyway, I think that at that particular time, if I could have had intercourse with that horse, with that old mare, I could have been able to separate the abstract from the concrete, the relative from the absolute, the cosmic from the uncosmic. I could have had friends. I could have belonged. I wouldn't be here today. . . . Well, I'm telling you that's what I think. I know it sounds stupid maybe, but that's what I think. . . . Okay. Thanks a lot. . . . Next week? In here, in your office? . . . Okay, thanks. Good-bye.

In the interchange just given, we are able to read only the words of the patient. He is adept at saying things that seem designed to startle the social worker. He makes frequent references to sexual thoughts and activities and admits to being "deranged" as he calls it. He lets the social worker know that he has been there long enough to have seen many professionals come and go. He seems to be subtly intimating that he is entering what he considers to be futile game of therapy because neither of them has a choice. He is giving her some bits of information to see how she will react so as to define the relationship that is beginning to develop between them. If he senses that he may have offended her or fancies that he has, he apologizes and tries to reestablish harmony. If he feels that she may be moving in too close as when she questions him about his mother, he changes the subject. These two individuals are beginning to form a basis for the information exchange which will be a pattern for their interactions for the next few days, weeks, or months. His "deranged behavior" controls the expectations and shifts the responsibility away from his tenuous self system.

Effect of Social Deprivation Since the social value of the digital data-processing system depends on constant synchronizing or tuning so that data are processed in a consensually validated fashion, we can speculate that social deprivation decreases the facility with which an individual utilizes this mode of data processing and data exchange. Clinically, this seems to hold true for psychotic patients who evidence difficulty in the analog-to-digital data-processing paradigm and in synchronizing their digital operations with others. The deficit produces isolation which, in cybernetic fashion, increases the deficit. This is particularly apparent when the individual is institutionalized for long periods. The chance of synchronizing the digital operation is decreased, resulting in more of a shift to the analog so that the patient may become more withdrawn or autistic. His digital operation becomes less synchronized, that is, his "associations become looser." His affect (emotional tone), stemming now from an unsynchronized analog-to-digital operation, is said to be "inappropriate."

Is the so-called inappropriate communication of the psychotic patient an attempt to define relationships, to set the expectations at the lowest common denominator as far as his own self system is concerned and thereby avoid the responsibilities required by those individuals who are synchronized with the world we term real? At present, we cannot answer this question. As long as the patient is able to drift in and out of the digitalization of programmable information, he will indirectly be in control (he controls by using behaviors that make others take control of him) and enjoy a type of security afforded by the institution.

Psychotic behaviors are perhaps the most frightening exhibitions of dissynchrony, and they are not as familiar as those symptoms termed *anxiety* and *depression,* which commonly disrupt family and other group information-exchange systems. There is usually no reason for the group members to institutionalize the anxious or depressed individual unless the individual is suicidal or abdicates reality testing. In our present culture, threatened suicide is often considered an acceptable reason to assume responsibility for another person's life. Families must cope with depressions and anxieties until they reach sufficient magnitude to warrant clinical and/or legal intervention.

Depression, Anxiety, and Anger

Depression is one of the most insidious symptoms of dissynchrony. It manifests itself in many different ways. Some of the more common signs of depression include crying, refusing to talk, withdrawing from the social and family group, losing all interest in previous activities, sitting and staring into space for long periods of time, losing or gaining weight, being indifferent to personal appearance, and appearing apathetic or overly worried.

The depressed person who claims to be unworthy of existence most often is not only communicating that he feels miserable, but is implying that this statement requires others to respond to the contrary. Depressed people may attempt to control the communication system and define relationships with others by derogating themselves. This safeguards them from criticism of others, implies that they are not responsible, decreases expectations, and often evokes supportive attention. Ironically, attention may reinforce depression as a coping technique.

If significant others agree that a depressed person is pitiful and feel sorry for him, he avoids responsibility for their response by stating he does not want pity. He thereby also avoids the responsibility for any anger or guilt that he evokes in others.

Depression may be effective in obtaining attention and may last until others fail to respond. The individual then must increase the tension by threatening suicide or by reversing the pattern and stating he feels better. The latter statement, being somewhat novel, draws attention. The better he feels the more attention he receives, until the family takes his state of well-being for granted and begins to divert their attention elsewhere. Then the individual must give signals of depression to draw attention again. This interaction may be related to the cyclic nature of depression.

The movement of an individual toward dissynchrony may be a cybernetic process with the early symptoms of dissynchrony being reinforced since these help the individual and his group to better understand his behavior. This is frequently seen in academic situations in which a student who becomes anxious is able to excuse low marks because of anxiety. This is not infrequently reinforced by understanding faculty who corroborate that the student is capable of much more efficient information processing than is apparent from the examination. The symptom of anxiety is now utilized as an explanation for not readjusting the self system's data-organization process. Consider the slippage of synchrony suggested in the following letter written by a student to her mother.

Dear Mom,
    We had our first final exam today and it was worse than a nightmare. We have our second exam tomorrow and I know I

should be studying but it's no use. I can't seem to concentrate. I read my notes but I can't remember what I've read. I have had difficulty in concentrating for the past month or so. I didn't mention it when I was home because I didn't want to worry you and Dad.

I know how much you are concerned that I get prepared for life but lately I am beginning to feel that I am not worthy of your trust and expectations. Several times last week while I was studying I found myself crying. I'm not sure why. I get angry at myself when I think how hard you and Dad have worked to give me this opportunity and I don't carry my part of the responsibility. It's gotten so when I take time out from my studies to go for coffee I feel that I'm an ungrateful wretch and that somehow I should be punished.

I do try to discipline myself. I have avoided any opportunities for dating this semester. I have stopped watching T.V. in the lounge and I haven't gone with the girls to a movie in over two months.

I made a "B" in chemistry test last week and I felt so ashamed I had trouble facing the professor the next day. My roommate tried to persuade me that a "B" is not a bad grade but she doesn't understand that with the opportunity I've been given it's like letting down all my friends and most of all, you and Dad.

Sometimes I feel I have wasted the most precious gift a girl can have—the love of parents like you. I am beginning to doubt that I am fit to have a place in life.

I am writing this to ask you please, please don't blame yourselves if I don't make it through the exams. You have done everything in your power and I love you more than anything else in the world. It is totally my fault if I let you down.

Your loving and unworthy daughter,

Pam

Pam is trying desperately to avoid what she feels are the expectations of her parents. She is defending herself by stating her efforts to do all she can. She is derogating her own self system and praising her parents, perhaps with the hope that they will lessen their expectations and feel guilty that she is suffering so much. She claims tremendous love for them and sorrow at her inability to live up to their examples. The emotions of affection that have been digitalized and paired with the word "love" have allowed this semantic unit to represent a conglomerate of analogical activity. This global abstraction includes feelings of insecurity, anger, and loss of self-esteem, resulting in the multivalent emotional state to which we have given the term *guilt*. Pam does what is so common in family "love" situations where the love is coupled with spoken and unspoken expectations. In return for the guilt she is feeling, she tries to evoke a similar guilt in her parents under the guise of being the suffering child who is too undeserving to exist.

The rage against the expectations of her self system and that of her family, which is usually present in guilt-laden exchange systems, has been veiled by her heavy emphasis on "love." One would not be surprised if this anger culminated in a suicide attempt, which would be a way of lashing out at expectations and simultaneously attempting to avoid responsibility.

Use of Dissynchronous Self System by Family and Community

In family organizations, information emitted from one of the family members that does not fit the prescribed and agreed-upon patterns that are acceptable to the family self system may be excused if the individual contends that he is not his actual self but suffering some affliction beyond his control, for example, headache or despondency. His complaints may draw more attention from family members than nonsymptomatic behavior, thereby reinforcing symptoms as efficient coping techniques. The child with a stomach ache may receive more attention from his parents than his sibling who attends school in a predictable fashion. This process is further complicated when the entire family self system under stress becomes somewhat dissynchronous. The anxiety of all family members may be allayed when one member is willing to accept his symptomatic behavior as the total cause of the family dissynchrony. Relief from diffuse anxiety may cause the family to lavish a great deal of attention on the individual who accepts the role of being the causal agent of family discord. This allows the family to establish a cause-and-effect relationship for its misery. This explanation temporarily smooths out the family communication system and increases the family synchronization by focusing on the dissynchronous behavior of one of its members. The sick role now becomes part of the family's data base for predicting its information-exchange system and maintaining its homeostasis.

Unfortunately, if the family communication system continues to be somewhat out of tune, the individual who accepts the sick role has to become more and more symptomatic in order to maintain the homeostasis. To paraphrase this concept, if illness in one family member is used by all the family to avoid responsibility for tension, the ill person's symptoms must increase when family may tension increases. Otherwise, the family might have to find another excuse. As that individual's self system is now set to program all data that validates him as a sick self, his flexibility and interpersonal skills deteriorate into a rather specialized communication system of anxiety, hypochondriasis, and depression. At this point, attempts to dissuade the sufferer from his role serve as a reinforcement, by increasing his anxiety and causing him to cling more tenaciously to this rationale for the deterioration of his interpersonal skills. Since the entire family may have become somewhat parasitic on this role in defining their own self systems, their interpersonal relationships with the symptomatic individual often reinforce the spiral.

In many families the utilization of one member as a sick role in the family self system provides a convenient escape mechanism or excuse when the family or members of the family do not meet the expectations of the community in which they live. In some families this escape mechanism may be of such convenience that several family members vie for the role of being the "sick one." This excuse may be used by all family members to prevent anxiety. However, the allaying of anxiety may diminish their drive to incorporate new information in the family self system.

Without the continual input of new information, the family self system and the individual self systems that compose it become more rigidified, stagnant, and impoverished until this highly specialized data-programming set can no longer negotiate in the information-exchange system at large. At this point the family and individual self systems become vulnerable to unprogrammable information from their social system. When this occurs, the family may pressure one of its individuals to seek help from a social institution or the community may pressure the family to search for more acceptable techniques of interacting. By extrapolation we may have a situation in which the community may use the "sick" family and the family may use the "sick" individual as an excuse for any disruption in their information-exchange system.

If the individual's symptomatic behavior causes him to contend that he is suffering, the family and community may select health institutions to address the symptomatology. If the individual's symptomatology causes others to suffer, the legal instruments of the social system be called into play. Since many patterns of behavior, including threatened suicide cause individualized and generalized suffering, both institutions may be involved so that the individual filling the sick role is forced to seek professional help.

Suicide as a Response to Expectations

An enormous amount of data have been compressed into an individual's chief complaint, "I am miserable." On further questioning, the individual may state that he has considered terminating his self system because it causes him misery and misery to significant others. Concealed within the statement "I am a burden to others" is its own antithesis, that is, "The expectations of others are a burden to me."

Self-destruction is an attempt to avoid the guilt arising from not fulfilling the expectations of a rigidified self system. The unrequitable expectations of this self system have been incorporated from the real or fantasied expectations of others and embellished by the individual in his attempts to achieve security. His search for security may include the acquisition of prestige and power, which paradoxically increases expectations and responsibilities culminating in more insecurity. Each acquisition that temporarily allays insecurity augments his love of self. The increased responsibility and expectations concomitant with these acquisitions may progress to almost constant frustration eventuating in self-hate. The guilt arises from a combination of self-love and self-hate and this irreconcilable antinomy may produce a fight–flight pattern with the flight pattern increasing individual isolation and further reifying self, and the fight pattern being directed at the punitive self system.

Suicide is an angry response to oppressive expectations. Kidnapping, blackmail, and murder are behavioral patterns that evoke anger and bitterness in most social units. Suicide is a behavioral pattern that contains similar elements and yet we respond differently. The threat to the life of a family member may be a conspiracy from outside the family or inside the family.

We choose to see suicide as a pattern of behavior for which no one is responsible except mental health professionals. We reinforce this pattern by ransom. If it were suggested that a program be set up whereby anyone considering skyjacking would receive immediate attention by dialing a number, we might decrease the number of skyjackers or we might, with enough publicity and concerned attention, increase the number of persons who utilize this pattern of behavior to draw attention to their frustrating life situations.

Should suicidal threats be the ticket for admission to health services? Or should the individual be advised that suicide is a coping technique that is optional but, if he wishes to explore other avenues, there are facilities available?

Suicidal rumination may reflect the need to escape a maladaptive self system derived from a dissynchronous analog-to-digital operation. The analog system does not function in the value judgments of the digital operation, since it does not differentiate into rigid categories of good, bad, right, wrong, stupid, or intelligent. However, it does respond to digital symbols as to any other input, and when the digital operation signals impending disaster the analog system responds with those emotions that would occur in the actual presence of danger. If these emotions become sufficiently intense, they decrease the efficiency of the analog-to-digital operation resulting in a cybernetic system of discomfort.

We may approach this system via (a) drugs to decrease or increase the state of arousal, that is, direct alteration of the analog-to-digital ratio, and (b) attempts to alter the digital operation by synchronizing it with digital operations that are more adaptive. The second may be futile since the digital operation is now so diminished by emotions from the analog system that all data processing is distorted. We may then attempt to alter the digital and analog systems simultaneously to achieve a more adaptive analog-to-digital ratio. In most cases, we increase the chances of successful realignment of the self system data base when we combine these approaches. By this conjoint approach, we may regulate the state of arousal by medication while we introduce the depressed individual to more productive communication techniques.

Anxieties, depressions, psychoses, and threats of suicide are all symptoms of the dissynchronous self system. These symptoms, which are a response to frustration, may paradoxically increase frustration in the individual and others. Symptoms often occur when the individual is unable to find other communication patterns that will give him stability. This paradox is compounded when the individual is so "undifferentiated" that he cannot accept even temporary separation from significant others in his reference group, even though the data emanating from the group increases his frustration.

For example, we often hear young adults complain bitterly about the oppressive tyranny of their parents even though they make no effort to leave home. This paradox is illustrated in the statement, ''I want to do my own thing'' subtly coupled with the unspoken statement, ''But I need my parents' approval.'' Or, ''My parents are stupid but I can't be happy unless they understand me.''

Differentiation   The term *differentiation* has been used to describe the flexibility of a given self system in processing data. By this abstraction we may indicate the individual's tolerance in accepting data that does or does not corroborate his self system and the intensity of his reaction to this type of information. For our purposes we will discuss three rather arbitrary categories of differentiation: (*a*) the overly differentiated, (*b*) the differentiated, and (*c*) the undifferentiated. The overly differentiated individual is self-locked, with all new information being screened by his rigidified self system allowing little contradictory data to be processed. The overly differentiated student might imply that any course he does not understand is ''irrelevant.''

The differentiated individual is aware of the relativity of his self system and how this self system influences his information processing. This flexibility allows him to negotiate a much broader range of informational input. He is able to use his self system as a working construct rather than as a finite entity and to shift its boundaries continually to incorporate new data. The differentiated student has the capability of admitting his lack of understanding and seeking help before passing judgment on course material.

The underdifferentiated individual has an unstable self system as his base of coding new data. His self system fluctuates so widely that each new set of information may cause disorganization and anxiety as he frantically attempts to reorganize his oscillating self-concept. The undifferentiated student expresses panic in every unfamiliar situation, implying that his peers are much better prepared than he.

The process of differentiation then becomes a continuum. The overly differentiated person exhibits inflexible patterns of behavior that may compromise his interpersonal skills and make him vulnerable to anxiety when data from his social system do not validate his rigidified set of ideas concerning himself. The underdifferentiated person is also vulnerable in that the rapid and labile shifts in his self-concept make his behavior unpredictable to himself and those in his social system. This hampers his interpersonal skills and decreases his ability to form stable relationships.

In the continuum from overly differentiated to under-differentiated self systems, the extremes have some similarity in that both produce insecurity with its concomitant symptomatology. This model of conceptualizing self systems on a continuum with underdifferentiation at one end and overdifferentiation at the other becomes complicated with the realization that a single self-concept may include elements from both extremes. For example, certain parts of an individual self system may be overly rigidified, whereas others are tenuous and flexible to the point of instability. The differentiated–underdifferentiated model may be a useful working concept for students of behavior if they keep in mind that these categories are arbitrary and a matter of degree rather than a matter of kind.

The underdifferentiated individual's behavior is often labeled hysterical. His behavior is extensively influenced by emotion from the analog system with less reliance on the linear logic of the digital operation. Interactions with others seem to lack predictability. His relationships seem quixotic, based more on "affect" (emotion) than on reason. He becomes insecure if other individuals are unable or unwilling to validate the rapid shifts in his self concept. The more anxious he becomes, the greater his shift toward the analogic computation of data. This increases the emotional component of his behavior, giving it a theatrical quality.

The overly differentiated individual's behavior is often labeled compulsive. He relies heavily on the digital paradigm. The intense reliance on his digital system may cause him to screen out information which is presented as emotion. Any stimulus that can not be digitalized results in a feeling of unpredictability, lack of control, and anxiety, with increased effort to digitalize the operation. As the anxiety increases, the individual may lock into a digital operation, that is, a compulsive or obsessive routine as a way of coping with a dissynchronized analog-to-digital flow of data processing.

Loneliness Evidence of dissynchrony permeates our cultural informational-exchange system. It is now difficult for an individual to be alone. Other persons are continually barraging our perceptive machinery with their presence and their communication via the media of spoken and written word.

The advent of television allows verbal and nonverbal communication to be transmitted directly into the home. Still, many people complain of feeling lonely. There is some indication that crowding may enhance this feeling. It has been speculated that the present flood of human communication depersonalizes or deemphasizes the importance of the individual self. It is also possible that crowded living and commercialized intimacy (for example, passive observation of television) precludes the dynamic interchange between the individual's self system and the self systems of others. The absence of this interchange may result in the individual's self system being narrowed and concretized into the role of nonparticipant observer.

Lack of participation prohibits the exercise of shifting self boundaries, leading to stultification of self-concept. This stagnation makes the individual self vulnerable to threats emanating from shifts in his social system. The vulnerability may lead to retreat, isolation, and deterioration of interpersonal skills, with further impoverishment in the information that makes up the self system.

The anxiety that arises from this frustrated information hunger may be temporarily allayed by the distraction provided by commercial media. This spiral may cause the individual self to atrophy until it become analogous to a parasite. It can no longer comfortably enter the information-exchange system of interpersonal relationships, but requires predigested information to satisfy its data hunger. Since the information obtained is incomplete, that is, lacking in the individual's participation, there is a residual unrequited feeling of hunger or emptiness that we term *loneliness*. The self system is the origin of loneliness in our crowded society just as it is the origin of all the other symptoms of dissynchrony.

Self-differentiation is one of the major attributes of the digital operation, and prevents the individual human from merging with the herd. We alluded to this phenomenon in Chapter 5, where we termed it *alienated dependency*.

The digital operation not only permits self-differentiation, it allows the realization that this differentiated self is finite, with a beginning and an end. Only the human self system, using the digital operation of which it is composed, can contemplate its own death. Death of the self and the concomitant fear of this inevitability seem unique to humanity.

Loneliness is compounded by our anticipation of not being. We may attempt to avoid this existential problem by involving ourselves with others. If we are unable to develop the necessary interpersonal skills for this involvement or allow our skills to deteriorate by observing without participation, we may experience an existential crisis.

The individual experiencing this type of crisis may become anxious concerning the meaning of his life and how he fits into the scheme of things. If our loneliness, insecurity, and subsequent dissynchronous behaviors cause sufficient discomfort to ourselves or others, we may seek or be brought to professional attention.

References

1. Forbus, W. *Reaction to injury*, Vols. I and 2. Baltimore: Williams and Wilkins, 1943.

2. Freedman, A., Kaplan, H., and Sadock, B. (eds.). *Modern synopsis of comprehensive textbook of Psychiatry/II*. Baltimore: Williams and Wilkins, 1975.

3. Kraepelin, E., *Manic-depressive insanity and paranoia*. Philadelphia: Saunders, 1973.

4. Marmor, M. and Pumpian-Mindlin, E. Toward an integrative conception of mental disorder in W. Gray, F. Duhl, and N. Rizzo (eds.), *General systems theory and psychiatry*. Boston: Little, Brown, 1969, pp. 297–309.

5. Szasz, T., *The myth of mental illness: Foundation of a theory of personal conduct*. New York: Hoeber-Harper, 1961.

Suggested Readings

Akiskal, H., and McKinney, W. Overview of recent research in depression. *Archives of General Psychiatry*, 1975, *32*, 285–305.

Arieti, S. (ed.). *Interpretation of schizophrenia*. New York: Robert Brunner, 1955.

Bleuler, E., *Dementia praecox or the group of schizophrenias* (translated by J. Zimkin). New York: International Universities Press, 1950.

Cancro, R., ed., *The schizophrenic syndrome*. New York: Brunner/Mazel, 1971.

Fabrega, H., and Ezeren, L., A behavioral framework for the study of human disease. *Annals of Internal Medicine,* 1976, *84,* 200–208.

Fair, C. *The dying self.* Garden City, New York: Doubleday (Anchor), 1970.

Farber, M. *Theory of suicide.* New York: Funk & Wagnalls, 1968.

Fischer, R. Hallucinations can reveal creative imagination. *Fields Within Fields,* No. 11, Spring 1974, Pp. 29–33.

Fischer, R. The perception–hallucination continuum. *Diseases of the Nervous System,* 1969, *30,* Pp. 1–11.

Flach, F. *The secret strength of Depression.* Philadelphia: Lippincott, 1974.

Hine, F., Pfeiffer, E., Maddox, G., Hein, P., and Fridel, R. *Behavioral science: A selective view.* Boston: Little, Brown, 1972.

Jackson, D. *The etiology of schizophrenia.* New York: Basic Books, 1960.

Mishler, E., and Waxler, N. *Interaction in families: An experimental study of family processes and schizophrenia.* New York: Wiley, 1968.

Pavlov, I. *Essays in psychology and psychiatry.* New York: Citadel Press, 1962.

Percy, W. *The message in the bottle.* New York: Farrar, Straus, and Giroux, 1975.

Pfeiffer, E. *Disordered behavior: Basic concepts in clinical psychiatry.* New York: Oxford University Press, 1968.

Sartre, J. *Essays in existentialism.* New York: Citadel Press, 1972.

Scheflen, A. Systems and psychosomatics. In W. Gray, F. Duhl, and N. Rizzo (Eds.), *General systems theory and psychiatry.* Boston: Little, Brown, 1969.

Snyder, S., Banerjee, S., Yamamura, H., and Greenburg, D. Drugs, neurotransmitters, and schizophrenia. *Science,* 1974, *184,* Pp. 1243–1261.

Toolan, J. Depression and suicide. *In* S. Arieti (Ed.), *American handbook of psychiatry,* Vol. II. New York: Basic Books, 1974, Pp. 294–305.

Suggested Questions

1. When may information be termed *dissynchronous?*
2. State two major categories of dissynchronous behavior.
3. Give a definition of *pathophysiology.*
4. Name one chemical agent that can be used to ameliorate dissynchronous behavior and one that might be used to produce dissynchronous behavior.

5. Give one danger of using chemical agents to escape anxiety.

6. Upon what is digital data processing heavily dependent?

7. What may happen to an individual who maintains a set of being ready to fight or flee?

8. What may happen to an individual whose attempts to realign his self system are continually thwarted?

9. Give one advantage of using the "response to injury" model when considering the classification of behavioral patterns.

10. State one way in which the categorization of behavioral patterns is helpful.

11. How may a state of panic affect the individual's ability to communicate?

12. Explain the ineffectiveness of platitudes in helping an individual.

13. Explain how institutionalization may shift expectations rather than give relief from expectations.

14. State one effect of social deprivation on the synchronizing or tuning of the self system.

15. Name some of the more common signs of depression.

16. Discuss interpersonal interactions as they are related to the cyclic nature of depression.

17. What may be the effect on family anxiety if one member is willing to accept his symptomatic behavior as the total cause of the family dissynchrony?

18. Discuss self-destruction as an avoidance phenomenon.

19. What need is reflected in suicidal rumination?

20. Give your opinion as to whether suicidal threats should or should not be the ticket for admission to health services.

21. State two ways of approaching the cybernetic system of discomfort. Give one deficiency of each approach.

22. Give three categories of differentiation.

23. Discuss the effects of decreasing the interchange between an individual self system and other self systems.

24. What are the concerns of an individual said to be experiencing an existential crisis?

10 Synchronizing Relationships

> Mammals in general, and we among them, care extremely, not about episodes, but about the patterns of their relationships. . . . This is crucial. This is what mammals are about. They are concerned with patterns of relationship, with where they stand in love, hate, respect, dependency, trust, and similar abstractions, vis-à-vis somebody else.
>
> Gregory Bateson, 1972(1)

Patterns of Relationships

With the evolution of the self and the growing dependency of each individual self system on other self systems, the human animal is enmeshed in patterns of relationships. These patterns are the center of his existence and, from birth to death, each person is engaged in a cybernetic system of information processing that validates his existence and adds to his illusion of autonomy.

Most individuals maintain a variety of relationships that have synchronizing effects. All these relationships are subject to discord or disharmony, depending on the type and intensity of the information exchanged. As we have discussed in previous chapters, all information has an effect upon the self system or self-concept. Most individuals are able to process information and make the necessary adjustments to their self systems. All persons have some discomfort in the maintenance of patterns of relationships but are usually able to keep a state of equilibrium or synchrony. However, as we illustrated in Chapter 9, some individuals are unable to make fine-tuning adjustments, and begin to emit dissynchronous behaviors. If the dissynchronous behavior continues to occur and/or increases in intensity, the individual self system may be brought to the attention of the therapist (professional synchronizer).

We are all familiar with such terms as therapist, therapy, and therapeutic techniques. People will sometimes comment that they have a "therapeutic relationship" with another person when they are signifying a type of friendship that they find beneficial in that it helps them to maintain synchrony.

Many students who begin their undergraduate studies in the biologic and sociologic sciences will eventually be in professions that are dedicated to helping other individuals maintain a state of equilibrium. They become adept in the utilization of information-exchange techniques that enable dissynchronous persons to regain sufficient control in their information-exchange systems to become and remain functional. These professionals form synchronizing relationships with those who seek their help.

Dissynchronous individuals who require professional attention are generally labeled *patients* or *clients*. The disadvantage of the use of these particular labels is that they also carry with them the idea of disease or illness, and may give the dysfunctional person a feeling of being "one-down" and/or the professional the converse feeling of being in a superior position. However, the term "patient" is so widely used that it is difficult to substitute another word. Therefore, we will continue to use the terms therapist and patient when referring to individuals involved in synchronizing relationships of a professional nature. However, we hope to broaden their definitions so that they seem less judgmental and stereotyped.

A Systems Approach to Disease, Illness, Normality, and Abnormality

Perhaps one of the greatest pitfalls for the beginning student of human behavior occurs with the introduction of such nebulous terms as *disease, illness, normality,* and *abnormality*. These concepts have biased students toward viewing people in diagnostic categories and in seeing variations in data processing as disease entities.

Anthony Reading has clarified some of the problems of integrating the psychosocial and biophysical approaches by more clearly differentiating between the concepts of illness and disease (4).

The sociologic sciences (for example, social work) have traditionally been seen as dealing more closely with illness if we accept Reading's definition of illness as "the patient's experience of ill-health" (4). The biological sciences (medicine, for example), on the other hand, have dealt more exclusively with disease which, according to Reading, "refers to various structural disorders of the individual's tissues and organs that give rise to the signs of ill-health" (4).

Perhaps the integration of the sociologic and the biologic sciences could be augmented by the deletion of certain terms including disease, illness, and, especially, mental illness. However, these terms have become so ensconced in public and professional vocabularies it seems more feasible to attempt to broaden and detoxify their usage.

Using the biosocial model, we might make the following statements:

1. Illness and disease are words used to denote abstractly a disruption of the synchronized relationship of intrapersonal and interpersonal systems.
2. Disease is a disruption of physiologic systems. Illness is a disruption of the way an individual conceptualizes himself.
3. Illness may arise from disease, a shift in relationships with others, or any factor that threatens the individuals. (For example, the depressions stemming from cancer of the pancreas or from family discord have some common denominators in neurochemical alterations, their behavioral readout, and the cybernetic disruption of individual and family relationships.)
4. Illness affects all systems to some degree and, therefore, affects the self-concept. (For example, a cut finger or a mosquito bite is a minor disruption of "me." A myocardial infarction—heart attack—or a divorce may represent a major disruption.)
5. Those system disruptions that have major effects on the individual's self-concept and its relationship to others have been termed *mental illness*.
6. Mental illness disrupts relationships in all internal and external systems including family and community.
7. The morbidity of illness and the effectiveness of treatment procedures is dependent on a synchronized approach to all related systems.

Despite efforts to use the terms illness and disease to denote abstractly dynamic shifts in various intrapersonal and interpersonal systems, the use of these terms always carries the liability of concretizing or rigidifying our thinking. They insidiously influence the users of these terms toward classifying activity within systems into normal and abnormal certainties.

The terms *normal* and *abnormal* have given us more problems than the terms disease and illness. As one of the authors of this book wrote several years ago in another text,

After differences are catalogued, the tendency is to group the individuals into categories labeled "normal" and "abnormal." While these may be useful terms for the researcher, they may be anathema to the clinician. The whole concept of normality and nonnormality is counterproductive for the clinician. . . . Normal, abnormal, bad, good, black, white—all these are judgmental and prejudicial terms that can cause the clinician numerous problems in dealing with patients who are obsessed with their own failures to conform [3, pp. 253, 259].

Although this particular text is not written strictly for the clinician in the health care fields but for the student of human behavior in any environment, the same observations hold true concerning the concepts of normal and abnormal.

The use of a systems framework in addressing human behavior allows the deletion of such concepts from our thinking. We see individuals not as normal and abnormal, but as interacting systems of data processing, interdependent and related, although diversified, in their methods of giving and receiving information.

This conceptual viewpoint may be difficult for students entering the health professions, particularly those in the field of mental health, who are confronted with a wide variety of theories concerning human behavior and with an equally impressive variety of therapies and techniques for addressing unproductive or dissynchronous patterns of behavior. Since physicians, psychologists, social workers, and counsellors perceive and communicate by a process of differentiation, emphasis is usually placed on the differences between the various therapeutic models rather than on their shared attributes. Scholars are often rewarded for innovative approaches, which influences them to elaborate more on the unique features of each new theory, leaving the student to weave all the theoretical frames of reference into some pragmatic pattern suitable to his or her own skills.

Synchronizing Techniques

In this chapter we will speculate on what we consider to be the lowest common denominator of therapy, rather than focusing on a particular set of techniques or media through which the message is delivered. We believe that the major differences among synchronizing techniques are in the methods or media of expression rather than in the basic information exchanged.

Most synchronizing techniques address, evaluate, and attempt to modify the information included in a person's self system, and how this coded information influences the individual's perception and behavior. Synchronizing approaches to the dissynchronous self system may range from shifting the state of arousal of the central nervous system to interpersonal manipulation via individual, family, or group information-exchange techniques. The major goal of any approach to synchronization is to help individuals evolve self systems that are in harmony with their own particular analog and digital data processing systems and that of others with whom they have contact.

The psychotherapy medium for addressing locked or distorted data-processing systems has multiple formats. The common denominator, whatever the specific format, seems to be an attempt to expand and realign the data base of the individual self systems involved.

Psychotherapy, then, is the synchronization of analog and digital operations and the addition of new information to the individual's self system, allowing a broader base for processing information from his environment. This realignment and addition of data may also provide more apparent options for emitting and responding to data. Psychotherapy may be thought of as a type of education. The evaluation of its effectiveness must, at present, be a pragmatic operation. The proof of its validity lies in whether or not the recipient shows greater efficiency in problem solving. The therapist or synchronizer must often rely on hearsay evidence to indicate whether or not the individual who has undergone a certain educational process is translating these data-alignment or problem-solving techniques into situations outside the therapeutic education system.

Forming Synchronizing Relationships

How, then, should the health professional approach an individual whose communication is out of synchrony with his own self system or that of others? The initial interchange between the professional therapist or synchronizer and the dissynchronous person (patient), like all other interpersonal relationships, is an information-exchange system. The therapist, through nonverbal and verbal communication patterns attempts to define a relationship with the suffering individual and significant others which allows the exchange of all pertinent data. If the suffering individual develops trust in the therapist and is not frightened by the expectations or judgmental attitude of the therapist, we state that the relationship is one of *rapport*. The development of rapport is dependent to a large degree on the therapist's self-control of nonverbal and verbal communications.

One of the first steps in evaluating the information-programming ability of the dissynchronous individual is the inventory of behavioral patterns and information concerning the onset of those patterns that are found disturbing by the individual and/or significant others. This inventory should include all of the interpersonal exchange systems in which the patient has been involved, especially those that immediately preceded the onset of dissynchronous behavior and those subsequent to the onset of this behavior.

Beginning students often attempt to study the behavior of an individual without inventorying the exchange system of his environment. It is important to examine the entire system because we are unable to state whether behavior is productive or nonproductive until it is seen in light of its exchange system. The individual self shifts continually, depending on the interaction with others. However, since many dysfunctional behavioral patterns have received intermittent reinforcement, they persist in new exchange systems for some time before being extinguished.

For example, a person who has grown up in a family situation in which he has been granted everything he wants and has been led to believe that he is always to have his own way, may expect the same treatment when he moves into a dormitory. He may exhibit outbursts of temper when "crossed" by his classmates. These outbursts are considered unacceptable and repulsive to his new peer group. Instead of getting his way through this method of expression, he succeeds only in alienating everyone. His discomfort may become so intense that he emits even more dissynchronous behavior and is referred to a professional for help. His behavior, although dysfunctional in his new exchange system, was quite functional in the old system. This information is vital to the professional who is attempting to establish a synchronizing relationship with this particular individual.

We are able to get some idea of the usual patterns of behavior an individual exhibits with others as he attempts to utilize these patterns in the exchange with the therapist. Unless the therapist is aware that he, too, is conditioned to exchange behavior in ways characteristic to him, he may label some behaviors as pathological because they are foreign to him and others as normal because they are familiar. He may not take into account whether or not these patterns are productive in maintaining a predictable relationship among individuals in the patient's environment.

Most textbooks of psychiatry and clinical psychology provide the student with a format for obtaining a history of present illness, past history, family history, social history, developmental history, and so on. Some of these texts fail to emphasize the effects that the communication patterns of the therapist will have on the data obtained. Some are weak in addressing the enormous influence of significant others in evoking and reinforcing various patterns of behavior we term dissynchronous.

Methods of Evaluation

The therapist should evaluate the patient's entire information-exchange system and approach the patient as a readout of a complex data pool in which information has been coded genetically and experientially from myriad contributing sources. Standardized instruments including the mental status examination and various psychologic tests can be used to ascertain the programming capabilities of the individual. With these instruments, standardized signals can be run through the individual's data-programming equipment and the readout compared with the average obtained from the responses of a large number of other individuals. This is particularly helpful in evaluating the efficiency of the individual's programming equipment.

Injury to the central nervous system or perceptive organs may impair an individual's ability to code information. These injuries range from acute toxic states produced by pharmacologic agents to actual destruction of brain tissues resulting from vascular insufficiency, neoplastic or infectious processes, metabolic derangements, or trauma. The physiological state of the entire organism must be considered in evaluating its programming capabilities. For example, individuals suffering from metabolic derangement or febrile conditions may have difficulties in programming information, and their behavioral readouts may appear distorted.

It should be emphasized that a limited capacity for digital operations does not necessarily preclude a productive and meaningful life style. There are many miserable people with IQs of 140 and many happy people with IQs of 80. It is probably the ability to form stable and rewarding relationships with others that makes the difference between these individuals.

Deciding What to Do   After completely inventorying the individual's history and programming capabilities, the therapist and patient enter the second phase of their partnership—"What is to be done about it." The initial goal of therapy is to help the patient arrive at a state in which he is able to program information at his maximum possible efficiency. If physiological disturbances impair this capacity, they must be addressed as quickly as possible by standard medical practices. If the individual is too panicked or despondent to participate in the inventory situations, pharmacologic agents may be utilized to alter his state of arousal to the optimal analog-to-digital ratio that we described earlier.

During the early stages of evaluation, the patient should be encouraged to participate in a one-to-one or a group learning situation in which his analog and digital communication patterns are synchronized with others. During the synchronization process, he is encouraged to digitalize or label his emotional state and exchange information concerning the effects that his communication patterns have on others, and vice versa. In this process, the patient may display patterns of behavior that have been reinforced by significant others, even though they seem to impair his ability to program new behavior and to communicate productively with others.

In the therapy situation, the patient is encouraged to digitalize as much information as possible concerning his interaction with others and to place this digitalized information in a logical sequence which will allow him to predict contingent information more efficiently. By this process of digitalization the individual is helped (a) to appreciate that this self system is a fluid working construct and (b) to add to the data base that makes up this self system. By broadening this data base and increasing the potential for programming new information pertaining to his self system, the individual may change his behavioral readout and become less vulnerable to information contained in the communication of others. This lessens the threats to his self system and thereby decreases his use of fight–flight patterns.

The Individual as a Group

In the relationship between a patient and a health professional, we have a situation analogous to the bumping of two icebergs. The information immediately available for the nonparticipating observer is only a very small part of the information influencing the interaction. The self systems of both individuals, the therapist and the patient, contain all of the information programmed genetically and experientially that we have described in previous chapters.

Both bring to the interaction patterns of communication and interpersonal skills that have been programmed from their interaction with individuals in the past. All of these past experiences are coded and referenced to one another. All the persons who have contributed to their respective information-exchange pools constitute an enormous group. Some of the group members imparted more information than others.

When the individual patient and therapist meet, there is an interface of these two enormous groups, with each group communication system being condensed into the communication system of each of the two participants. How the relationship will be defined and the type and quantity of information exchanged between these two depends on (a) the communication skills of each and (b) the information stored in the memory banks of each. Theoretically, the therapist should have a broader bandpass or tolerance for accepting information, and a more flexible way of rearranging data than the patient, whose suffering emanates from a rigidified or disorganized coding paradigm. It is the patient's nonflexible self system that interferes with his analog and digital coding apparatus, impairing his interpersonal skills and his potential for acquiring and programming new information. Therapists are not immune to this type of deficit.

Since "self" is in large part a working concept evoked from and for group interaction, it may be addressed as a group phenomenon. It contains group interactions, parental and family programs stored in memory banks. Two self systems interchanging information may be seen as two groups negotiating. Berne has called these negotiations "transactions" and breaks each self into three components—parent, child, and adult—representing roles or patterns of behavior utilized in defining relationships (2). A child may play the role of parent to his parents who play the role of child.

It is not sufficient for the individual to receive information. He must participate in the information-exchange system. Therapy is this participation. The "patient" may realign his self system as he gives and receives information in a mutually agreed upon learning paradigm.

Both self systems are driven by information hunger, which results in a type of searching behavior for information that will validate their respective self systems and allow the predictable coding of future information from their environment. This searching behavior is influenced by an attitudinal set of expectations that each individual derives from his self system and that of others. The individual whose self system has incorporated the role of therapist includes in his self system the expectation that he can utilize his data bank to evaluate the data bank of others. By using his own coded information, the therapist attempts to help the patient realign his data so that he, too, can develop a more predictable coding system. The subsequent behavioral readout of this altered coding system may help the patient participate more productively in the information-exchange system of his family and community.

Importance of Mutual Understanding

The key concept in this description of therapy is centered upon the phrase, "mutually agreed upon." Often, the beginning therapist (a medical student, for example), certain that he is progressing along therapeutic avenues that will "work," assumes that the patient is willing to follow him along the same pathway. The agreement is understood only by the student, who becomes provoked when his advice is not followed. The following is a short and perhaps exaggerated illustration of what can happen between a student therapist and a patient when the agreement is not clearly understood.

THERAPIST: Good morning. Are you feeling better?

PATIENT: Not really.

THERAPIST: Why not? Didn't you do what I told you?

PATIENT: I tried but it didn't work.

THERAPIST: I don't think you are trying hard enough.

PATIENT: Tell me again how to do it.

THERAPIST: You just have to let out all that bottled up anger. Express how you really feel.

PATIENT: I don't know how.

THERAPIST: Come on. Try, tell me how you really feel about me.

PATIENT: I'm afraid you'll get angry.

THERAPIST: Don't be silly. You can trust me. Let it out. How do you really feel?

PATIENT: O.K. I'll tell you, Doc. I think you're a smug little son-of-a-bitch who thinks he knows everything. I think you don't understand me and are more interested in my money than anything else. You never listen to what I have to say and I'm sick and tired of your trying to run my life. What's more, I . . . .

THERAPIST: Hold on. You're getting upset. You don't really feel that way. You're just displacing your feelings about your family onto me. Can you see that?

PATIENT: God damn it, you bastard, there you go again, always changing things around.

THERAPIST: I can see you're still very tense and anxious. I think we ought to increase your medication.

PATIENT: Maybe you're right. I'm sorry.

THERAPIST: Now you take two of those orange pills at bedtime instead of one. When you get calmed down, we can talk more about how you handle your feelings.

PATIENT: Thanks, Doc. I'm sorry about popping off.

THERAPIST: That's OK. I understand you're still not yourself. See you tomorrow.

PATIENT: Thanks again. Goodbye.

In the preceding vignette, it would have been difficult for the patient to realign his self system, as there was little consistency between what the student said and the way he behaved. All the patient could do was say the "right" things and keep the student from being too upset. So long as the student could give advice and have it followed, he felt secure until the advice he gave, that is, "Let all your feelings out," was followed and turned out to be more than the student could assimilate into his own data-processing system at that particular time. When he began to lose control of the situation, he immediately fell back to the one-up role of doctor, prescribing an in-increase in medication. The patient followed the verbal and perhaps the nonverbal signals and again adopted the submissive role required by this particular therapist. There is a paradox in the way in which the relationship was defined. The therapist indicated he was in control and would give advice, and the patient would follow the advice. The therapist shifted this agreement when the patient, obeying his command, gave information that threatened the therapist's self-concept. The new therapist-imposed agreement states, "Obey my commands—in some situations but not in others." This patient would probably hesitate to follow any directions that encouraged the expression of his feelings toward the student therapist, who showed that he was unwilling to program this type of information.

The Need to Help Others or to Seek Help If the therapist is somewhat insecure in his role as therapist, he may be under pressure for information that will validate what he and others expect of his self system. He may need information from his clients or patients that validates his role of therapist, which is another way of saying that he may need to help others. This need on the part of the therapist to help will influence the interaction between therapist and patient in three areas:

1. The way in which the relationship is defined.
2. The control system involved in the relationship.
3. The type of information that will be exchanged.

The patient who has been pressured by his own insecurities or those of his family or community to assume the role of sufferer or help seeker may give a double message. He may (a) overtly express his need for help but (b) covertly be reluctant to give up behavioral patterns and attitudinal sets that have allowed predictability in his relationship to others.

It is worth emphasizing again that the relationship that will evolve between the therapist and patient is under the pressure of expectations from within *and* without, and these expectations will influence the information-exchange system that will be negotiated in their interaction. These expectations, which are in themselves coded information, have been referred to by the analytic school as the *transference* and *countertransference* phenomena. Information that does not immediately fit with the expectations of either individual will be programmed with difficulty, or resisted. If the nonsyntonic, that is self-disruptive, information is of sufficient quantity or quality and the pressure resulting from the needs of the therapist or patient to have the other party program this information are of critical magnitude, both parties may exhibit fight–flight patterns ranging from anger to withdrawal. In the patient–therapist interaction, the relationship is controlled by the self system that requires the least attention in maintaining a homeostatic relationship with its environment.

The therapist who has a great need to help in order to maintain his self system may require a patient to give him attention and information that validates his role of helper. Conversely, the patient who is attempting to avoid the anxiety resulting from meeting expectations may seek to avoid responsibility for his behavior by presenting information that indicates he is the victim of forces beyond his control, whether they emanate from fate, family, or community.

The therapist and patient may reach an impasse when (a) the patient assumes an attitudinal set of passivity and/or irresponsibility and (b) the therapist assumes an attitudinal set of desiring control but feeling too insecure to assume responsibility. The following is an example of a student therapist's ambivalent attempt to make a relationship complementary.

THERAPIST: Do you really think you are God?

PATIENT: Yes.

THERAPIST: How do you account for your thoughts on this matter?

PATIENT: They are not my thoughts.

THERAPIST: Not your thoughts?

PATIENT: No, I have no thoughts.

THERAPIST: Could you elaborate on that?

PATIENT: I do not exist as a person. As God, I am everything.

THERAPIST: Then who would you say I am talking with?

PATIENT: You do not exist.

THERAPIST: What is going on here and now?

PATIENT: Here does not exist; here is everywhere. Now does not exist; now is always.

THERAPIST: How would you go about proving such a statement?

PATIENT: There is no need of proof.

THERAPIST: I don't understand.

PATIENT: Proof is a phenomenon of logic based on differentiation. When there is a realization that all is God, the need for proof does not exist.

THERAPIST: Who realizes this abstraction?

PATIENT: God is the only reality.

THERAPIST: And you are God?

PATIENT: Yes.

THERAPIST: Then I am talking to God?

PATIENT: No, you are God.

THERAPIST: So God is talking to God. Is that what you are saying?

PATIENT: If you understand it better that way.

THERAPIST: Wait a moment. You just implied that I understand. Doesn't that imply a separate existence for me?

PATIENT: In one frame of reference.

THERAPIST: So you admit there are two frames of reference?

PATIENT: No, not two, infinite numbers or one, one and all are the same.

THERAPIST: This is an impossible argument, don't you think?

PATIENT: Yes.

THERAPIST: Why do you argue but refuse to follow any logical frame of reference?

PATIENT: I am not arguing.

THERAPIST: Don't you realize this is a commitment procedure and that I have the power to institutionalize you?

PATIENT: You may choose to institutionalize us both but you have no power over me since you and me are illusions.

THERAPIST: Don't start on that again.

PATIENT: All right.

THERAPIST: Now, tell me, do you think you can drop all this nonsense?

PATIENT: Certainly.

THERAPIST: Then you don't really believe you are God?

PATIENT: No, I am not God.

THERAPIST: That's better. Maybe if you take your medicine you will be able to remain in the community but it is necessary for you to stay on your medicine or otherwise you will start on this delusional kick about God. Do you understand?

PATIENT: Yes.

THERAPIST: Now that you have admitted that you are not God, can you tell me why you must be on medication?

PATIENT: Because you say so?

THERAPIST: Not because I say so. Because you need it.

PATIENT: You are not responsible for my needing it?

THERAPIST: Of course I am not responsible for your needing it.

PATIENT: Then who is responsible?

THERAPIST: You are responsible.

PATIENT: Am I responsible for deciding I don't need it?

THERAPIST:	No, you are not able to make that decision.
PATIENT:	Who makes that decision?
THERAPIST:	I make that decision.
PATIENT:	Then you are responsible for deciding that I need medication.
THERAPIST:	Yes.
PATIENT:	How did you arrive at that decision?
THERAPIST:	From my education.
PATIENT:	What was educated?
THERAPIST:	My brain.
PATIENT:	Where did your brain come from?
THERAPIST:	From a fertilized ovum with a genetic template that evolved over millions of years from molecular interaction.
PATIENT:	Where did the molecules come from?
THERAPIST:	Hell, how do I know? You're wasting time. Let's just say it's a God-given fact.
PATIENT:	Would you say I came from a God-given fact?
THERAPIST:	I don't care what you say. Just take your medication or you'll end up in the state hospital.
PATIENT:	One God-given fact would put another God-given fact in the state hospital?
THERAPIST:	If you like to think of it that way.
PATIENT:	Do you like to think of it that way, Doctor?
THERAPIST:	I don't like to think of it at all. I only do what society demands.
PATIENT:	Am I in society?
THERAPIST:	Not for long if you keep blowing your mind with abstractions. Don't think so much. Just go along with society.
PATIENT:	Just let my "self" go, like letting myself merge with God, only I should call it society instead?
THERAPIST:	Perhaps that would be better.
PATIENT:	You're saying then that you and I don't really exist. Only society exists.
THERAPIST:	I see where you're going with your schizophrenic logic, and I warn you, you're going to end up in the hospital. Just take your medicine and stop thinking so damn much.
PATIENT:	Thank you, doctor. I appreciate our time together.
THERAPIST:	You're welcome. See you again in two weeks.

Both parties attempt to control the relationship by abdicating responsibility for the information exchange.

The therapist attempts to control the relationship by making society responsible for his information. The patient avoids being controlled by preventing a delineation of his self system.

Effects of Therapist Assuming Responsibility

In therapeutic relationships, as in other interpersonal exchange systems, insecurity on the part of the participants may result in attempts at control while simultaneously avoiding responsibility for the information exchanged. In a more clearly defined complementary relationship, the therapist accepts total responsibility for the relationship and the patient accepts no responsibility for the relationship. Superficially, it would appear that the therapist has assumed control. However, his need to help leaves him extremely vulnerable and dependent on the patient to give him information that validates his role as helper.

On further scrutiny, we can appreciate the control techniques of the patient in that he lets the therapist assume the position of responsibility only so long as the therapist does not exhibit expectations that the patient accept part of the responsibility for their interaction. By allowing the therapist to assume responsibility the patient forces the therapist to (*a*) validate his (the patient's) role as irresponsible patient and (*b*) shield him from the expectations of others. The information exchanged in the interaction of patient and therapist is limited by the definition of helper and helpless, so that data emanating from either party is biased to prevent threatening the self system of the other. This continuous and mutually self-serving relationship may be sustained for extended periods if the therapist and patient agree to focus on information that does not mandate renegotiation of their relationship.

The development of a helper–helpless type of relationship is usually detrimental. Even though it alleviates symptoms of anxiety, at the same time it evokes a tremendous dependency from the client or patient. If the health professional sets himself up as the expert and helps the patient to solve the immediate problems at hand, he may be inadvertently short-circuiting the patient's ability to learn to cope with future problems. The patient then becomes dependent on the therapy situation, and at every stress returns to get answers. This makes the professional feel needed, wanted, and loved. It also gives the patient a feeling of security, resulting in his becoming an appendage of the professional's self system rather than attempting to develop a more differentiated data base.

It is very difficult for the beginning therapist to see an individual suffering from various patterns of behavior without moving in to take over and superimpose his own problem-solving techniques on the individual. This is usually not successful, since the environment that the professional lives in is not the same as that of the patient, and the solutions may be nonproductive, or, in some cases, augment the difficulty.

A focus for information exchange that usually proves nonthreatening to both participants concerns persons and situations somewhat removed from the relationship between the two, the patient's history. Many hours can be spent in inventorying the patient's previous experiences, during which the patient can present quantities of information stored from childhood that justify his present state of irresponsibility. By giving attention to this information, the therapist demonstrates that he is a caring individual, and the patient's gratitude for his concern corroborates his role as a helper. This mutually self-serving relationship (*folie à deux*) may go on at intervals for several years, with little change in either individual. One individual uses his patient status as part of his self system to ameliorate expectations from himself and others. The other individual has his role of helper validated by the attention of the patient evidenced by his return week after week. In most cases, the therapist pays more attention to the patient than the patient pays to the therapist and this deficit is made up by the patient in terms of money which is, in itself, an abstract form of attention.

If the therapist's self system is very secure, he may subtly shift the responsibility for the relationship into a partnership and, by mutual scrutiny of the interpersonal techniques that go on between the two, broaden the data base of both self systems involved in the therapeutic endeavor. In the latter situation, therapy becomes a type of learning laboratory in which both parties exchange information that will enhance their communication skills and increase the flexibility with which they exchange information with others.

The skill with which the therapist directs this learning interchange or controls the relationship is directly dependent upon the amount of information and type of information he has stored in his self system. The therapist who learns a broad range of interpersonal skills and who is aware of the needs emanating from his information hunger will be less vulnerable and less subservient to his need to be needed.

Recognizing the Needs of the Therapist

The realization that the therapist has needs that are constantly fluctuating is usually the most difficult and important concept for the student therapist. If he fails to program this concept, his own unrecognized needs may distort his response to the needs of others. If he sees himself as a helper of humanity or a helper of individuals that are in various states of misery, it may become necessary that those individuals respond to him in such a way that he feels like he is needed and that he has helped them or cured them. If, after his initial efforts, there is no improvement, or little improvement or change in the patient's patterns of behavior, his own need for seeing himself as a competent professional may be threatened. He then may begin to exhibit patterns of behavior that more and more reflect his own needs rather than those of the individual he is trying to help. He may become angry at the patient who contends he has not been helped. Since he wishes to conceptualize himself as a kind, understanding professional, he may deny that he is angry even though this anger biases his communication and jeopardizes his relationship with the client or patient.

The following illustration demonstrates the anger of a beginning therapist who becomes more and more frustrated with the interchange as the patient resists his attempts to "help."

THERAPIST: Tell me how I may be of help to you.

PATIENT: I tell you, they are out to get me.

THERAPIST: Who are they?

PATIENT: I don't know. Probably some combination of the CIA or FBI.

THERAPIST: Do you really think you are that important?

PATIENT: No, but they must. Since they are out to get me.

THERAPIST: They are not out to get you.

PATIENT: Did they tell you they're not out to get me?

THERAPIST: No, they didn't tell me.

PATIENT: How do you know then?

THERAPIST: I know, because this is one of your delusional systems.

PATIENT: What's a delusional system?

THERAPIST: A system of beliefs that you get out of your own head with no proof.

PATIENT: Like your knowing they're not out to get me?

THERAPIST: You're being passive aggressive.

PATIENT: What's passive aggressive?

THERAPIST: That's when you're angry but won't admit it.

PATIENT: Are you angry at me?

THERAPIST: No.

PATIENT: Are you being passive aggressive?

THERAPIST: No, now stop arguing with me.

PATIENT: I'm sorry.

THERAPIST: Now what seems to be the problem?

PATIENT: They're out to get me.

THERAPIST: You're trying to be difficult.

PATIENT: What do you want me to say?

THERAPIST: I want you to look at what's bothering you.

PATIENT: They are bothering me.

THERAPIST: You don't want help, do you?

PATIENT: Yes, that's why I'm here.

THERAPIST: Then why don't you try to make sense?

PATIENT: I am trying to.

THERAPIST: Perhaps you don't trust me.

PATIENT: I do trust you.

THERAPIST: Then believe I am trying to help you.

PATIENT: O.K., Doc. Do you trust me?

THERAPIST: Yes.

PATIENT: Then believe they are out to get me.

THERAPIST: It's plain to see you do not want help. You want your stupid delusional system validated. Don't blame me if they don't give you a pass to go home.

PATIENT: Who are they?

THERAPIST: The staff that decides who goes home and who doesn't.

PATIENT: Are they working for the CIA?

THERAPIST: For Christ's sake, it will serve you right if they keep you here forever.

PATIENT: You think they really are out to get me?

THERAPIST: I've been trying to help you, but you're wasting my time. Goodbye.

The patient in this vignette is quite adept at leading the beginning therapist in circles and refusing to follow his admonitions. The therapist falls into the trap of using professional phrases and trying to explain them to a person who is probably already well versed in the terminology and able to direct the interchange accordingly. For example, the patient seems to see the anger of the therapist who denies it. The therapist, in frustration, attempts to place the responsibility for the futility of the discussion on the argumentative patient. In this particular exchange, the student therapist finally becomes angry enough to disrupt the conversation and disengage himself from a situation that is proving too threatening to his own self-concept as a "helping" person. His anxiety at the impending loss of control results in a behavioral pattern similar to that of the patient in that he projects responsibility onto an omnipotent "they."

We have focused on the need to be needed or the need to help as major stumbling blocks for the beginning therapist. This is an irony in that this need may be one of the major motivating forces in causing the student to enter the health professions.

This need is also the cause for a large number of patients being labeled "crocks" when they express their frustration in hypochondriacal symptoms. Since their symptoms cannot be validated by laboratory data as stemming from physiologic disturbances, the student may be caught in a bind. The patient may deny emotional problems and the laboratory may disclose no physiologic problems, leaving the student frustrated in his need to help. The bitterness arising from this frustration may compromise his involvement with the patient and result in the self-protecting conclusion that the patient is a "crock." The term implies that the patient is unwilling or unable to play the doctor–patient game by the prescribed rules.

The student should keep in mind that he brings other needs and judgmental attitudes to the therapy situation. He may "like" or "dislike" patients because they remind him of other persons who have threatened or validated his self-concept.

Individual, Family, and Group Therapy

The therapeutic learning paradigm that is limited to the therapist and patient has some assets and some liabilities. One asset is the possibility for intense emotional investment between the parties, which may prove extremely effective as a model for learning more productive skills in intimate relationships. The intensity of the relationship may also be a liability in that the fulminating dependency needs of one of the participants may surpass the needs of the other, resulting in an impasse. This impasse may in itself prove to be a learning situation, or it may result in sufficient anxiety to terminate the interaction.

The relatively recent emphasis on family and group psychotherapy has resulted in the evolution of learning laboratories, in which multiple self systems are directly involved. In this type of therapy, several therapists and several patients may interact, expanding the social validation system in which behavioral patterns are inventories. In this type of group interaction, whether the members be family or unrelated, the focus is usually on the verbal and nonverbal readouts of the individual self systems and how these behavior patterns affect each participant's relationship with other individuals and the group as a whole. In these multiparticipant learning situations there is the opportunity for multiple definitions of relationships. An individual may define his relationship as authoritative to one member of the group, subservient to another member, symmetrical to another, and so on. Although these multiple definitions usually occur in individual relationships, the behavioral readout of these definitions appears to be more sequential in the one-to-one interaction, whereas their concomitance is more evident in the group interaction.

Since the individual has to define his relationships simultaneously with several individuals in his social system, the group model has the advantage of more closely resembling the community in which the patient lives, and thereby may make the learning experience more translatable into his everyday life. The pressure that a group exerts on one of its members to adjust his patterns of behavior depends upon the cohesion of the group, that is, the emotional investment each member places in the group as an organization or system of behavioral validation. This cohesion may be catalyzed by the individual participant's sharing with other group members emotionally laden information that he considers crucial for the maintenance of his self system or a potential threat to his self system. As this information is shared among group members, the group develops what might be termed a group self system, which gradually sets tolerance limits on the behavior emanated from the individual self systems. The synchronization of communication emanating from the individual's self system gives the group and the individual greater efficiency in predicting response patterns, and, hence, a feeling of security and belonging.

In the group process, individual dependency needs are usually diffused among several group members rather than focused on an individual therapist. This may decrease the potential for rejection. However, when the entire group refuses to validate certain patterns of behavior, the individual is under greater pressure in some respects in that he cannot excuse this type of rejection as being an idiosyncrasy of an individual therapist.

Entire families may be involved in the therapeutic process, since the distorted behavior in one member of the family may distort or be a response to a distortion in the behavior of other family members. Taking inventory of the whole communication system within a family or having the individual explore his communications system and feeling states in a group of other individuals who also have problems has proven to be extremely productive for learning other patterns of behavior. This is sometimes painful, but it may provide a more lasting ability to solve problems. This is sometimes quite difficult for the health professional since it may be easier to set up a one-to-one relationship, where the therapist can control the situation and feel that he is important as a problem solver. In family and group therapy situations, the catalyst for change is more diffuse.

Elevated Emotional States Returning to our crystal metaphor, we may state that the cognitive knowledge of a given individual is a crystal of digitalized units of information surrounded by a solution of analogically coded information, including emotions and instincts. There is a dynamic interaction between the solution and the crystal. If the emotional state is elevated, the crystal tends to dissolve, with recrystalization when the emotions subside. This is similar to Pavlov's experience with dogs that had been conditioned or taught a certain pattern of stimulus–response sequences. When a flooding of the laboratory caused extreme anxiety in the dogs they "forgot" their learned patterns, that is, their crystallized sets were dissolved by emotion (5).

This phenomenon has been utilized by individuals involved in "brainwashing." Sargent, in his book *Battle for the Mind*, describes how the ideational or cognitive set of an individual becomes more vulnerable to realignment if his emotional state is elevated to high levels of fear or anger (5).

In group interaction, the insecurity of the individual self is accentuated by a barrage of new information from others. If he develops a high pitch of emotion he may, at least temporarily, realign his whole conceptual set, as has been seen in religious rituals and revivals. Whether the new patterns persist depends on the reinforcement paradigm of his environment.

Group and family therapy can result in a change in the individual's relationships to others. If the entire family is involved, there is more likelihood of reinforcement of new and, it is hoped, more productive patterns than if the individual attempts to evoke reinforcement responses from family members who have not participated in the learning program and may be threatened by a shift in his behavior. They may respond in the manner that was standardized prior to therapy. These conditioned responses from others, which do not reinforce new behavior, may cause rapid extinction of the new behavior and a return to the previous behavior that "fit" the response.

Much has been written discussing the various forms of therapy and their merits and pitfalls. It is our belief that the success of different therapies and counseling, regardless of the techniques used, hinges on the information exchanged.

Therapy as a Learning Paradigm

In our discussion of therapeutic relationships, we would like to emphasize the following concepts:

1. Therapy is a pattern of learning. This occurs through relationships in which information is exchanged. The manner of establishing relationships is contingent on data emitted and processed by two or more individuals. The relationship is a cybernetic exchange of data, which differs in each relationship. However, the general pattern an individual utilizes in establishing relationships may have certain characteristics, depending on his data base, especially data relating to the self system stored from previous experiences. In psychotherapy, an inventory is taken of this mode of operation.

2. In the therapeutic relationship an inventory should be taken of the individual's programming capabilities. If his state of arousal is outside the range of efficient learning (for example, panic or coma) or if the individual's programming equipment is disrupted (by, for example, neoplastic, ischemic, or infectious processes), phar-

macological or physiological intervention may be necessary to obtain the optimal analog-to-digital ratio for learning.

3. Therapy is broadening the data base of the self system and tuning the analog and digital data-programming system within the individual and between the individual and others. Increasing the databank that pertains to the self system may help the individual appreciate the relativity of self and thereby increase his flexibility in consuming self-qualifying information from others.

4. In all therapeutic relationships there is the development of expectation sets called transference and countertransference. The patterns utilized in other important relationships become apparent in the relationship between two or more individuals. Evaluation, that is, putting the information in these patterns into a digital format allows a more linear and predictable data arrangement. This process may help the individual to become aware of behaviors that result in unproductive or disturbing cybernetic patterns and to substitute more effective behaviors.

5. *Insight* is the programming of old data from the digital and analog systems into a new sequence of digital data that allows greater flexibility in coding new information, particularly that which has reference to the self system. This realignment is therapeutic if it enhances the individual's capacity for participating in the information-exchange system of his family and community. The process of acquiring insight may, according to Freudian theory, involve "making the unconscious conscious," which may be paraphrased into "making analogic data transformable to the digital coding system."

6. The professional who deals with emotional problems must continually inventory his own self system. The behavior emanating from his "self" is the major tool he uses in addressing the problems of others. It is grandiose to assume that these tools will fit all problems. He must understand that his tools often require sharpening and occasionally become antiquated. He must be willing to borrow tools from others and to discard those tools that are no longer effective.

7. The desire to help others may be a covert expression of the need to be needed. Satisfaction or frustration of this need may distort the therapeutic relationship.

8. A paradox may arise when the beginning student attempts to evaluate "objectively" other humans' behavior. Since the data obtained usually result from an interchange between the observed and the observer, to maintain an "objective" stance, the data arising from the observer's participation is excluded from the digitalized conclusions. This causes limitation and distortion of the student's concepts about the behavior of others. It is mandatory, therefore, that the student appreciate the subjective data (his input) as being as important as the objective data (the patient's input).

References

1. Bateson, G. *Steps to an ecology of mind.* New York: Ballentine, 1972, p. 470.
2. Berne, E. *Principles of group treatment.* New York: Oxford University Press, 1966.
3. Porterfield, P. A clinical approach to the theoretical constructs of failure and normality. In N. Datan and L. Ginsberg (Eds.), *Life-span developmental psychology: Normative life crises.* New York: Academic Press, 1975.
4. Reading, A. Illness and disease. *Medical Clinics of North America,* 1977, *61* (4), 703–710.
5. Sargent, W. *Battle for the mind.* Hammondsport, England: Penguin Books, 1961.

Suggested Readings

Ackerman, N. *Psychodynamics of family life: Diagnosis and treatment in family relationships.* New York: Basic Books, 1958.

Arieti, S. (Ed.), *American handbook of psychiatry,* Vols. I, II, III. New York: Basic Books, 1974.

Benton, A. Psychological tests for Brain damage. In A. Freedman, H. Kaplan, and B. Sadock (Eds.), *Comprehensive textbook of psychiatry/II,* Vol. 1. Baltimore: Williams and Wilkins, 1975.

Bowden, C., and Burstein, A. *Psychosocial basis of medical practice: An introduction to human behavior.* Baltimore: Williams and Wilkins, 1974.

Carr, A. Some instruments commonly used by clinical psychologists. In A. Freedman, H. Kaplan, and B. Sadock (Eds.), *Comprehensive textbook of psychiatry/II,* Vol. 1. Baltimore: Williams and Wilkins, 1975.

Enelow, A., and Swisher, S. *Interviewing and patient care.* New York: Oxford University Press, 1972.

Forbus, W. *Reaction to injury,* Vols. 1 and 2. Baltimore: Williams and Wilkins, 1943.

Freedman, A., Kaplan, H., and Sadock, B. (Eds.), *Comprehensive textbook of psychiatry/II*, Vols. 1 and 2. Baltimore: Williams and Wilkins, 1975.

Gazda, G. *Basic approaches to group psychotherapy and group counseling*, Springfield, Illinois: Charles C Thomas, 1968.

Haley, J. *Strategies of psychotherapy*. New York: Grune and Stratton, 1963.

Havens, L. *Approaches to the mind: Movement of the psychiatric schools from sects toward science*. Boston: Little, Brown, 1973.

Hollender, M., and Wells, C. Medical assessment in psychiatric practice. In A. Freedman, H. Kaplan, and B. Sadock (Eds.), *Comprehensive textbook of psychiatry/II*, Vol. 1, Baltimore: Williams and Wilkins, 1975.

Jacobs, A., and Spradlin, W. (Eds.), *The group as agent of change*. New York: Behavioral Publications, 1974.

Kadis, A., Krasner, J., Weiner, M., Winick, C., and Foulkes, S. *Practicum of group psychotherapy*, 2nd ed. New York: Harper and Row, 1974.

Kraepelin, E., *Manic-depressive insanity and paranoia*. Philadelphia: W. B. Saunders, 1973.

Langs, R. *The technique of psychoanalytic psychotherapy*. New York: Jason Aronson, 1973.

Lieb, J., and Slaby, A. *Integrated psychiatric treatment*. New York: Harper and Row, 1975.

MacKinnon, R. and Michels, R. *The psychiatric interview in clinical practice*. Philadelphia: W. B. Saunders, 1971.

Mead, G. The i and the me. In T. Parsons, E. Shils, K. Naegele, and J. Pitts (Eds.), *Theories of society: Foundations of modern sociological theory*, Vol. 1. New York: Free Press, 1961.

Nagy, I., and Spark, G. *Invisible loyalties: Reciprocity in intergenerational family therapy*. New York: Harper and Row, 1973.

Oppenheimer, H. *Clinical psychiatry: Issues and challenges*. New York: Harper and Row, 1971.

Roeske, N. *Examination of the personality*. Philadelphia: Lea and Febiger, 1972.

Rosenbaum, C., and Beebe, J. *Psychiatric treatment: Crisis/clinic/consultation*. New York: McGraw-Hill, 1975.

Ruesch, J. Communication and psychiatry. In A. Freedman, H. Kaplan, and B. Sadock (Eds.), *Comprehensive textbook of psychiatry/II*, Vol. 1. Baltimore: Williams and Wilkins, 1975.

Sager, C., and Kaplan, H. *Progress in group and family therapy*. New York: Brunner/Mazel, 1972.

Spradlin, W. Family roles of the elderly as a focus in teaching comprehensive medicine. *The Journal of Medical Education*, 1966, *41* (4).

Stevenson, I. *The diagnostic interview*. New York: Harper and Row, 1971.

Szasz, T. *The myth of mental illness: Foundation of a theory of personal conduct*. New York: Hoeber-Harper, 1961.

Weinstein, E., and Kahn, R. *Denial of illness: Symbolic and physiological aspects*. Springfield, Illinois: Charles C Thomas, 1955.

Yalom, I. *The theory and practice of group psychotherapy*, 2nd ed. New York: Basic Books, 1975.

Suggested Questions

1. Under what conditions might an individual be brought to the attention of a therapist?

2. Give a disadvantage of the use of the labels *patient* or *client*.

3. How have the concepts of disease, illness, normality, and abnormality biased students?

4. Give one definition of disease. Give one definition of illness.

5. How does use of a systems framework in addressing human behavior permit the deletion from our thinking of such concepts as normal and abnormal?

6. What is the major goal of any approach to synchronization?

7. Give a definition of psychotherapy.

8. When can a relationship be said to be one of rapport?

9. Why is it important to inventory the entire exchange system of an individual who is asking for help?

10. Why are such standardized instruments as the mental status examination and various psychologic tests used?

11. What is the initial goal of therapy?

12. State two ways in which an individual is helped by the process of digitalization.

13. Give two factors that have bearing on how therapeutic relationships will be defined.

14. Discuss "self" as a group phenomenon.

15. Give three areas in which the need of the therapist to help will influence the interaction between patient and therapist?

16. Explain the "double message" that may be given by a patient who has been pressured to assume the role of sufferer.

17. Which self system controls the relationship in a patient–therapist interaction?

18. Give two conditions under which the therapist and patient may reach an impasse.

19. Discuss what happens when the patient allows the therapist to assume responsibility.

20. Discuss the detrimental aspects of a helper–helpless type of relationship.

21. What is usually the most difficult and important concept for the student therapist?

22. Give an asset and a liability of the therapeutic learning paradigm that is limited to the therapist and patient.

23. Give an advantage of the group model.

24. What happens to the cognitive set of an individual if his emotional state is elevated?

25. Discuss two of the eight concepts which the authors emphasize in their discussion of therapeutic relationships.

11 Cultural Coding Systems

All nature is a continuum. The endless complexity of life is organized into patterns which repeat themselves—theme and variation—at each level of system. These similarities and differences are proper concerns for science. From the ceaseless streaming of protoplasm to the many-vectored activity of supranational systems, there are continuous flows through living systems as they maintain their highly organized steady states.

James Grier Miller, 1978 (1)

Human Group Dependency

In the early phases of our evolution, it is probable that we associated with other humans in a manner resembling a wolf pack or a troop of chimpanzees. In this type of social structure communication among individuals in the group is largely analogic in nature, consisting mostly of nonverbal signals and vocal expressions of emotion that contain little in the way of abstraction.

As we evolved the capacity and acquired the skills for digitalizing information and the interpersonal sharing of this information via language, our social structure began to resemble more that of social insects. The similarity between the human social system and that of social insects is rather superficial, but both systems have become dependent on informational codes. In insect societies, the social code appears to be genetically programmed, whereas in human societies, only the potential for socially coding information is inherited, with the actual coded program being implanted in the individual by the social system in which the person lives. In both of these systems the individual is dependent on the group, with different individuals performing different functions for the group so that the function of the group is different from that of any of its individual units.

At present, our dependency on the group appears to be somewhere between that of the loosely associated wolf pack, in which each individual is totipotential, and that of the insect (for example, bees or termites), in which the individual cannot survive outside the group structure.

Importance of Digital Operation

In the previous chapters, we have addressed how the individual evolves a self system by use of the digital operation, which allows differentiation from the environment. We have referred to groups of these individual self systems that may share information to form an operational construct we termed the family self system.

Through this conglomeration of coded information, which we call the family self or family myth, individuals synchronize their behavioral patterns and communication skills and evolve a system of expectations for each of the family members, with each one assuming a graded responsibility for the family self system. We would like to transpose this model onto larger groups, which we will call the *social system* or *culture*, and which may include many individuals and families. The social self is obviously a metaphor. The individual self is also a metaphor, although not such an obvious one.

The cohesion of a social self system is dependent on its digital operation for coding information. Just as in the cell colonies that we described in an earlier chapter, whether or not a social system evolves and survives is dependent on the efficiency and flexibility with which it processes information. If its coding system is too general, the system may lack the cohesion and efficiency necessary to program routine data, in that all of its members are more or less totipotential, with a great deal of redundancy in their activities.

Dangers of Group Specialization

As the individual units specialize and share their information with other individuals who have differing specialties, the efficiency is markedly increased. If the group becomes overspecialized, its efficiency in programming routine data may preclude the introduction of new information, leaving the organization obsolete if there are marked changes in its environment.

The study of history gives us a number of examples in

which cultural systems became dominant through their efficiency in handling certain types of information. As the systems became rigidified, they screened out new information, leading to stagnation and decay.

The decline of these societies may be in part due to the overspecialization of a system or coding pattern within the organization, since the social organization, like the multicellular organism, is composed of numerous systems for data processing. These systems contain roles that are analogous to the roles that make up the individual self system. We may arbitrarily delineate some of these systems as agricultural, religious, legal, military, medical, political, academic, and economic. All of these systems within the greater social system are concerned with acquiring information and aligning this information in such a way that data coming from future events fall within predictable boundaries.

Rules, Ethics, Morals, Laws

Using these data-processing systems, the social self evolves expectations and responsibilities like the individual self system. These are mediated through information sets we may term *social ethics* or *laws*, which define the relationship of the social self system to the self systems of its members. These rules or patterns are expected to maintain a predictable relationship.

Often, the social self is termed a *state* or a *nation*. Occasionally, it is personified as illustrated in the posters throughout America a few decades back stating, "Uncle Sam Needs You" and portraying a social self system as an elderly man with white whiskers and a top hat pointing at all who passed. This objectification was perhaps the result of the digitalization of information and our ability to differentiate "self" from the environment. We then apply the subject–object dichotomy to all relationships, including the social self, of which the individual self is a cybernetic part. Having accomplished the illusion of individual autonomy, we are confronted with the problem of digitally coding the relationship to the larger self system and to the unknown in a manner that allows us to predict future data. These two major cultural relationships are concretized in the phrase "For God and Country." The attitudinal sets of these relationships, whether they be termed religion or patriotism, often overlap. For example, it would be difficult to distinguish attitudinally the religious fanatic from the patriotic zealot. The rules, ethics, or morals for defining the relationship between the individual and social self, are often attributed to a reified abstraction—God or country.

The rules that regulate patterns of behavior especially those concerning sex, aggression, property, and the rights of others are sometimes attributed to the state, and at other times to one or more gods. Those who are unwilling or unable to abide by these socially validated regulations may be labeled sinners and/or criminals.

If social regulations or expectations become dissynchronous with the information programmed in a sufficient number of the individual self systems, the laws are changed, either by common consent or revolt. Occasionally, ethics and expectations are altered by religious leaders, prophets, or messiahs.

Religious Systems   The individual's adherence to the rules of the state is encouraged by threats to person and property. Our cathexis to a religious ethical system, often a covert instrument of the social self, is catalyzed by our awareness of the transient nature of our self systems and our fear of the unknown. This fear, coupled with our information hunger, results in a shifting mixture of affective tone including loneliness, anxiety, awe, and reverence. We are driven by this multivalent emotional state to negotiate a working thesis for understanding the interface between ourselves and our perceived nonselves. Our floundering attempts to digitalize the operation have led to many fascinating word sets that have been referred to as myths.

These myths are mechanisms for concretizing the unknown into delineated entities, that is, deities, good and evil forces, and so on, that allow us to conceptualize a cause-and-effect relationship between events we vaguely perceive in ourselves and our environment. To call these working constructs "myths" seems very appropriate if we understand that the individual self system also fits this description. It may be cogent to speculate that these religious or cultural myths are the multiple extensions and reflections of the self myth which, as we have reiterated, is a technique for information coding.

Religion may be humanity's earliest attempt at the abstract exercise of explaining, and, even though it at times appears rather crude when scrutinized by modern logic, it contains the enlaga or precursors of those activities now so highly prized as art and science.

These latter are refined techniques of data arrangements emanating from the same source and still containing many elements of religion. What artist or scientist can eliminate the feeling of awe and insecurity in the face of the unknown? The elimination of this attitudinal state would probably reduce dabbling with data to a rather technical activity, and would probably preclude the imaginative or intuitive realignment of information that produces new concepts or new ways of understanding relationships. Our stereotyped actions would lack the drive for newness that we call creative.

We may state that much creativity then was initially expressed in behavior we would call religious. If the system established by this religious behavior sufficiently allayed information hunger and insecurity about relationship to the unknown, it may have been digitalized into ritual and standardized formulas called dogma that inhibited further investigation.

Scientific Systems   Science, the child of religion, continually rebels against the stultifying arbitrary boundaries set up by its parent. As science comes of age there are signs that it, too, is delineating boundaries that exclude information-processing systems like metaphysics. There is fear that metaphysical speculation will be concretized into a dogmatic system as often occurs in religion. However, in setting metaphysics as "off-limits" for science, there is the paradoxial evolution of scientific dogma.

Many scientists indulge in metaphysical speculation secretly and are ashamed if this activity is found out by their colleagues. If the speculation bears fruit in terms of more productive data-processing operations, the credit is given to imagination, intuition, or serendipity. Newton is said to have indulged in metaphysical speculations about numerology and even dabbled in alchemy. However, he adamantly separated these activities from his scientific observations.

The reader might do well to address any system of information coding, whether it be religion, art or science not as good or bad, right or wrong, but in terms of its efficiency in coding data and its flexibility in allowing new data to assimilate with or counteract data already programmed. Systems that inhibit this can be labeled dogma, whether they be in religion, science, or art.

The religion, art, and science now prevalent in most cultures in varying combinations are techniques for moving information from the analog coding system to a digital coding system. Technology evolves when digitally coded information is standardized into formats that seem of pragmatic value to the cultural system.

Efficiency of Language

The digital operation of a social system is dependent on the instruments used. We have addressed the use of language when words are paired with digitalized units of information. The efficiency of language as an information-coding instrument varies among cultures.

The development of a flexible alphabet as opposed to pictographs and the evolution of integers 0–9 as coding systems gave enormous flexibility to the digital data-processing system. It appears that cognitive sets and philosophy follow in the wake of the particular digital paradigms used to code data. Since all digital operations are based on differences and contrasts, the highly developed digital operations of the Western societies emphasized dualistic thinking or the subject–object differentiation prominent in Aristotelian logic. This pattern of information coding lends itself well to technology, as has been evidenced in Western societies since the Renaissance, culminating in the Industrial Revolution.

In the last few thousand years, since humans have been able to digitalize and record their digital efforts, we have seen a phenomenal advance in technology. The resultant technological equipment has enhanced our digital operation so much that we can now, by the use of instruments, further segmentalize and differentiate or compartmentalize our environment.

Perhaps the most significant advance attributable to this digital operation is the vast increase in communication techniques. With the elaboration of electronic media, digitally coded information is rapidly shared with many members of the human species. Computer technology has allowed this information to be stored in large quantities with efficient retrieval of enormous sums of data. We must keep in mind, however, that this is only quantitatively different from the data recorded in hieroglyphics stored on clay tablets.

The digital operation is also apparent in architectural endeavors, with the biggest advance coming when we learned to digitalize or unitize building blocks from which we created edifices bearing no resemblance to the unit or building block itself. When we moved from caves and mud huts, which were of analog design, to domiciles built of individualized units, the process of digitalizing information was well on its way. It must be emphasized that the phylogenetically older analog system is still a major coding paradigm. The synchronization, or integration, of the analog and digital processing systems is not yet complete.

We still have trouble digitalizing all of the physiological processes that go on within us, including emotional states, innate drives, and instincts. This vast array of information that cannot be digitalized and put into the word paradigm of a self system is said to be *unconscious*. That these unconscious or analog processes have an effect on our relationship to our environment and social system is quite apparent to any student of human behavior.

Effects of Technology on Data Processing

One of the paradoxes of modern Western societies may stem from the effect technology has on data processing. Until recently, communication patterns were heavily oriented toward digitalized data favoring science and technology. Most mass communication was exchanged through the written word. Technology has allowed new media for transmission of information including telephone, motion pictures, radio, and television.

The telephone has permitted individuals to communicate over large distances, allowing vocal intonations of analogic derivation to influence the communications more than was possible in letter writing. Television gives even greater emphasis on analogically coded nonverbal data.

A child no longer has to translate from the digital medium to conceptualize a knight in shining armor on a snow white steed. The knight can be visualized directly on the screen. The information moves in analogic fashion from the observed to the observer. This may, in part, explain the drop in IQ of school children, since "intelligence" is usually an indication of skill in handling digitalized data. The child now can get the analogic picture without practicing translation to and from the digital code.

Thus, technology, the product of digital data processing, seems to be decreasing the digital coding skill by presenting information in analogic form, and partially eliminating the need for digitalization.

Regardless of the communications media, we still must negotiate the relationship between our individual self systems and the social self system. This relationship always contains the phenomena of expectations and responsibility.

Social Responsibility and Legal Systems

The question of social responsibility poses many problems. Various theories assert that the individual has always been and will always be the victim or benefactor of his genetic and social heritage. The person's behavior emanates from the dynamic interaction between one's external milieu and the genetically programmed substrate of one's physiology.

With this method of conceptualizing human behavior, it follows that no one is responsible for his or her own behavior. We are by no means masters of our destiny, for who selects our parentage and who selects the social milieu of our childhoods? An ancient reference states, "And which of you with taking thought can add to his stature one cubit? If ye then be not able to do that thing which is least, why take ye thought for the rest?" (Luke 12:25, 26). This philosophical set might lead to the assumption that human interaction is unpredictable.

Biologists might protest by postulating genetically determined templates or innate behavioral regulators, and sociologists contend that social pressures and group dynamics have evolved predictable systems for regulating human behavior. It is in this quandary between social regulation and preprogrammed genetic heritage that we come to the impasse now confronting professionals in the field of health and those in the field of law.

The scientific students of behavior, being aware of the numerous contingencies that influence the readout of the organic computer we call the human central nervous system are reluctant to endow any individual with total responsibility for his or her action. On the other side of the dilemma, legal professionals contend that no social system can operate without a system of rules predicated on individual responsibility and arbitrarily agreed upon by the group in which the individual lives. Although the rules may be renegotiated periodically, owing to shifts in group needs, without some format or code of conduct the human social unit would be in a continual unpredictable state of flux.

It was probably early in our social evolution that we assumed the "as if" proposition that each of us is responsible for our own activity. In earlier cultural systems those people who transgressed social codes of conduct were labeled as guilty and punished according to specified regulations.

This archaic social system of guilt and punishment persists, even though we are now able to conceptualize abstractly social rules as instruments for protecting society rather than as weapons for revenge. This anachronistic duality of punishment and protection has led to social guilt for punishing individuals whose behavior indicates that they do not have the ability to maintain the stance of responsibility. In order to avoid the guilt of punishing someone who is not responsible, we have gone to great lengths to differentiate between those who are and those who are not responsible, even though responsibility was initially, and continues to be an arbitrary phenomenon or an "as if" proposition.

Certainly, society cannot operate without the illusion of individual responsibility. Yet, scientific evaluation of human behavior might reach a dead end if it assumes the same philosophical set. It is this impasse that has caused heated debate between professionals dedicated to the study of individual human behavior and those involved in studying the instruments of social regulation.

Although lawyers continually request help from behavioral scientists in differentiating between those individuals who are responsible and those who are not, they are often disappointed by the nebulous responses. Perhaps this impasse could be bridged to some degree by the realization that the two sets of professionals are working out of different paradigms. It seems unproductive to argue about which paradigm is better since both are necessary but mutually exclusive.

It would be helpful in negotiating differences between the two systems if behavioral scientists could better appreciate the need for instruments of protecting society while the legal profession was given a better view of the philosophical sets of the behavioral scientists.

The chasm between the two systems is broadened by the professional narcissism prevalent in both camps, resulting in each boasting a more complex overview of the total human situation. The issues are further confused by ambivalence in society as to whether legal instruments are protective or punitive.

It has been suggested that if we were able to discard the punitive aspects of law enforcement, and look upon laws as instruments for protection of the social self, then individuals might be seen in a relative continuum of being more or less dangerous to society rather than being either responsible or not responsible for their activities.

With this format for conceptualizing human behavior, our penal institutions could move to educational and rehabilitational programs for those individuals who need to learn better techniques for relating, and humane detention centers for those individuals who have given indication that they will be dangerous to society for a prolonged period. This would eliminate the category of criminally insane, allow all parties to maintain the dignity of the "as if they were responsible" position, protect society, and, at the same time, give a path of reentry into society for those individuals whose behavior placed them in opposition to the social structure.

This sounds very humane. However, the danger lies in the phrase "protection of society." Protection might mean screening out all information that threatens society or brings about change. It would be easy to utilize the "protection of society" motif to incarcerate dissonant individuals, decreasing the input of new information. There are indications that this now occurs in some societies. The solution to the problem may lie in a more flexible social system rather than the rigid system that evolves when information input is distorted or inhibited.

The need of the social self system for rules to regulate the behaviors of its individuated units has also resulted in the evolution of various educational systems. Through education, individual self systems can be taught, not only the information deemed desirable by the social self, but the professional roles which are necessary for the propagation of the social self system.

Educational Systems The values of any particular culture in the more digitalized or industrialized nations are reflected in their educational systems. For example, since human life is considered sacred in Western society, the education of physicians is thought to be of paramount importance, and the competition for entrance into medical school is almost overwhelming. Status and security for the physician are at such a high level that the profession of medicine is believed by many to be the ultimate. Medicine lends itself easily to social approval because it satisfies not only the desire of the individual self to achieve and to help mankind but it reifies the social self by trying to assure its longevity. Through faith in medicine, man may attempt to avoid his mortality.

As the Western culture becomes more technological, there is an increased demand for specific knowledge and for such professions as engineering, computer programming, mathematics, and physics. The social self demands that all its needs be met and those needs are, to a great extent, linked with the products of technology, for example, television sets, automobiles, computers, and air conditioners.

The emphasis on technology may indicate an imbalance in the social self by the hypertrophy of one of its information-processing systems. By hypertrophying one of these systems, a social organization may become transiently more efficient in data processing than those surrounding it, but this hypertrophy may subsequently lead to disharmony with other systems in the organization and subsequent decline of the organization. If, for example, the religious system of a culture becomes dominant, its techniques for coding information concerning the unknown may allay anxiety of the individual members of the culture, increase the cohesiveness among the individuals in the cultural system, and instill a fervor and dedication in the culture which allows it to become a dominant influence over other cultures. If this religious organization begins to exclude any new or unprogrammable information that it considers threatening, the culture may become vulnerable to other cultural systems that are more flexible and able to program information that enhances their efficiency.

Similar situations can be seen in cultures that focus on military prowess, bureaucratic political systems, or even artistic, scholastic, and economic endeavors. For those in academics it would seem that this system is the least pernicious in that its major emphasis *is* the programming of new information. Yet, if the majority of the members of a cultural system were involved in this activity without addressing information concerning the aggression of surrounding cultures, an academic society might be overrun by a culture that had placed emphasis on an older type of information—that associated with military skills.

As our information pool has increased, we have also expanded our technological capabilities so that this information now permeates most of the leading cultural systems. Rapid dissemination of digitalized information has, to some degree, broken down the barriers that isolated cultural systems a few hundred years ago. Unfortunately, under stress, individual cultures still emerge as isolated units and show many of the fight–flight patterns that we have seen in the individual who becomes dissynchronous with his group. A good example is the fight–flight patterns of the Third Reich in the 1930s and 1940s, in which an entire nation exhibited paranoid and aggressive tendencies with catastrophic results stemming from emphasis on the military system.

Behavioral Patterns in Societies

It would seem that societies utilize the same behavioral patterns as individuals in attempting to ameliorate the anxiety generated in periods of stress or by situations that do not lend themselves to closure. For example, social selves or nations may undergo depressions or elations (periods of boom) or they may become paranoid. This paranoia may be grandiose or persecutory ("We are the master race," "That territory belongs to us," "They are out to destroy us"). If this attitude persists, the social self may resort to an aggressive method of handling its anxiety. War may be the method of attempting validation or relief.

What causes group anxiety? We may speculate that it is generated by a coming together of individual anxieties. When enough individuals in a social system do not feel their roles are sufficient to provide security and predictability of the future, the conglomerate feeling becomes that of being out of control. Just as individuals abdicate responsibility for this behavior, groups can also deny responsibility (for example, consider lynch mobs and riots). If the group attempts to establish security by screening out dissynchronous information, the individual who presents disruptive information may become the enemy of the social self (consider Galileo or Martin Luther King).

Social Self Systems

Social systems are analogous to the crystalline relationships of units. As a system crystallizes, it aligns the information of its units and the alignment becomes information which forces the units into place. The development of a social self is the predictable relationship of the individual self systems which then incorporate the social self into their self systems. This cybernetic pattern may be disrupted by pressure from dissynchrony within the individual self system, the social self system, or both.

The social self is a data-processing instrument that

allows prediction of data from within and without and is subject to threats. It may be loose and general, or specialized. The more specialized, the greater the temporary efficiency. If the external environment shifts, the greater the possibility that the specialized social self may become obsolescent.

The social self is an "as if" paradigm, as "real" and relevant to human existence as each individualized self system. This conglomeration of individual self systems termed the social self has its own autonomy and acts upon things and reacts to events as predictably as the individuated self.

The social self is most differentiated in periods of stress, for example, national crises such as war or the assassination of a leader. During a time of conflict, patriotism is a cohesive attitude, which binds most of the individuated self systems into the social self system. When a popular leader is assassinated, the social self grieves and may become righteously indignant and determined to retaliate against the killer or killers.

Not all periods of cohesion are associated with tragedy or violence, but most are probably associated with an elevated emotional state in the majority of individuals in the social system, resulting in the illusion of oneness. This can be seen during holiday periods, for example, Hanukkah, Christmas, and Thanksgiving, when individuals speak of the holiday spirit, the feelings of good will and harmony. At these times, our search for synchrony seems to culminate in a unified effort which serves to alleviate our anxiety and allow us to deny our individual mortality or to disguise it so that it appears less frightening.

Just as the individual's search for synchrony and information hunger generate self-esteem, the social self seeks its own reason for being. The bicentennial celebration in the United States emphasized the birth of a social self, its differentiation from a mother culture, and its emphasis on democracy as its *raison d'être*.

Like the individual self, the social self systems may realign their data-processing patterns before the discord becomes symptomatic. There is some indication that Western cultural patterns are now shifting. Despite the emphasis on technology, there are growing counterforces arising from a type of information hunger that technology has not been able to satisfy. There is an increased awareness by the social self of a threat to its existence because of the misuse of natural resources and an awakened international interest in ecology and its related professions.

During the past century, the boundaries between Eastern patterns of data processing, which do not emphasize the subject–object dichotomy, and the elite digital operations of Western cultures seem less distinct. This may be due to Western emphasis on the relativity of such data-processing concepts as time and space. As our theories about the space–time grid upon which most dualistic thinking has been plotted become more flexible, the arbitrary nature of subject–object differentiation becomes evident in our data-processing systems. This has resulted in a decrease in the rivalry between religion, art, and science. Perhaps this indicates a broadening of the data base that makes up the social self and an increase in the potential for incorporating new data. Perhaps it indicates a regression to a more analogic type of data programming. Natural selection may decide its efficiency.

Summary   Through biologic and social evolution, the human being has become a specialized animal. The specialty is the digital coding of data. That this specialization, temporarily at least, favors survival is evidenced by the enormous number of people now living on this planet.

Other animals have specialized—the dinosaur, the saber-toothed tiger—all with a temporary increase in survival efficiency followed by extinction. Our specialty has allowed us to process more information than any other animal. This information has allowed self-differentiation with concomitant fear of anticipated death and suffering and the development of a social self, again with differentiation and global wars.

The digital system has allowed technology, producing terrifying instruments of destruction, various types of pollution, and consequent disruption of the Earth's ecosystems. These developments have led some to suggest our return to a more simple analog system similar to other animals. However, we are committed and cannot give up our digital operation any more than the saber-toothed tiger could absorb its fangs. Perhaps a marked shift in the environment and an alteration in the present natural selection may result in a different type of person, but this will take eons.

Our hope lies not in abdicating the acquisition of information but the intensification of this process. We must acquire enough information to become aware that our self-referencing systems and all the data we program are relative.

Reference 1. Miller, J. *Living systems*. New York: McGraw-Hill, 1978, p. 1025.

Suggested Bazelon, J. D. The perils of wizardry. *The American Journal of*
Readings *Psychiatry*, 1974, *131*, 12.

Bronowski, J. *The ascent of man*. Boston: Little, Brown, 1973.

Durkheim, E. On sacred objects as symbols. In T. Parsons, E. Shils, K. Naegele, and J. Pitts (Eds.), *Theories of society: Foundations of modern sociological theory*, Vol. II. New York: Free Press, 1961.

Durkheim, E. Religion and society. In T. Parsons, E. Shils, K. Naegele, and J. Pitts (Eds.), *Theories of society: Foundations of modern sociological theory*, Vol. I. New York: Free Press, 1961.

Durkheim, E. Society and individual consciousness. In T. Parsons, E. Shils, K. Naegele, and J. Pitts (Eds.), *Theories of society: Foundations of modern sociological theory*, Vol. II. New York: Free Press, 1961.

Edwards, P. (Ed.). *Body, mind and death*. New York: Macmillan, 1964.

Fromm, E. *The forgotten language: An introduction to the understanding of dreams, fairy tales and myths*. New York: Grove Press, 1957.

Halleck, S. Legal and ethical aspects of behavior control. *The American Journal of Psychiatry*, 1974, *131*, 4.

Lanternari, V. *The religions of the oppressed*. New York: Mentor Books, 1965.

Malinowski, B. On the social functions of religion. *in* T. Parsons, E. Shils, K. Naegele, and J. Pitts (Eds.), *Theories of society: Foundations of modern sociological theory*, Vol. I. New York: Free Press, 1961.

Miller, J. *Living systems*. New York: McGraw-Hill, 1978.

Piaget, J. *Insights and illusions of philosophy*. New York: World Publishing Company, 1972.

Richards, O. *The social insects*. New York: Harper Torchbooks, 1961.

Toynbee, A. The disintegration of civilizations. In T. Parsons, E. Shils, K. Naegele, and J. Pitts (Eds.), *Theories of society: Foundations of modern sociological theory*, Vol. II. New York: Free Press, 1961.

Trivers, R., and Hare, H. Haplodiploidy and the evolution of the social insects. *Science*, 1976, *191*, 249–263.

Watts, A. *Psychotherapy east & west*. New York: Ballantine Books, 1969.

Weber, M. The social psychology of the world religions. In T. Parsons, E. Shils, K. Naegele, and J. Pitts (Eds.), *Theories of society: Foundations of modern sociological theory*, Vol. II. New York: Free Press, 1961.

Suggested Questions

1. Compare human societies and insect societies with regard to the coding of information.

2. The evolution and survival of a social self system is dependent upon what factor?

3. Discuss the danger of group specialization.

4. Discuss one or more situations that might result in the changing of laws.

5. What factors catalyze our cathexis to a religious ethical system?

6. Describe one way in which technology evolves.

7. How are the data stored in computers different from the data stored on clay tablets?

8. Discuss the possibility that technology may be decreasing the digital coding skill.

9. Discuss some of the differences between theoretical frames of legal professionals and behavioral scientists.

10. Give one reason why medicine lends itself easily to social approval.

11. What causes group anxiety?

12. Compare a social system with the crystalline relationship of units.

13. Describe the social self.

14. What is the specialty of the human being?

15. In your opinion, does the digital operation increase or decrease man's chances of survival?

12 Evolution of a Systems Theory of Self and Society

It is no easy matter to study social phenomena in the only right way—viewing each element in the light of the whole system.

Auguste Comte, 1896(9)

. . . social evolution forms a part of evolution at large.

Herbert Spencer, 1898(18)

Direction of Thought Toward Systems

Wherever human societies have existed, there have been those who have theorized about the individual self and about the dynamic interaction between each person and his culture. While it was not practical to attempt an examination in this book of all theories of the individual and society, it is crucial to note that there seems to be an evolution of thought in the direction of viewing man as a set of systems within larger systems.

We are becoming more aware of the cybernetic relationship between individual and social systems. The importance of the dynamic interaction between the individual and his culture was recognized fairly recently as a result of the efforts of scholars from many disciplines.

We will, in this chapter, give a brief overview of some of the concepts that have evolved over the past 400 years concerning the relationship of man to his cultures. Figure 12.1 is not complete, but it does present some of the foremost scholars who have addressed concepts concerning man and his environment and indicates the direction our present theories seem to be taking. The selection of those theorists who represent the different areas of study

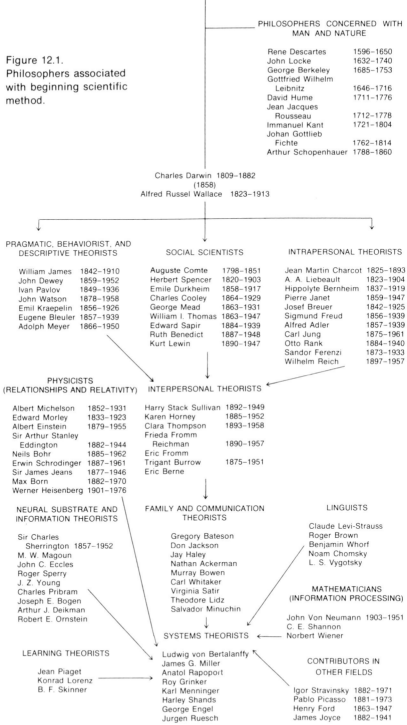

Figure 12.1.
Philosophers associated
with beginning scientific
method.

Francis Bacon 1561–1626
Thomas Hobbes 1588–1679

PHILOSOPHERS CONCERNED WITH
MAN AND NATURE

Rene Descartes	1596–1650
John Locke	1632–1740
George Berkeley	1685–1753
Gottfried Wilhelm Leibnitz	1646–1716
David Hume	1711–1776
Jean Jacques Rousseau	1712–1778
Immanuel Kant	1721–1804
Johan Gottlieb Fichte	1762–1814
Arthur Schopenhauer	1788–1860

Charles Darwin 1809–1882
(1858)
Alfred Russel Wallace 1823–1913

PRAGMATIC, BEHAVIORIST, AND
DESCRIPTIVE THEORISTS

William James	1842–1910
John Dewey	1859–1952
Ivan Pavlov	1849–1936
John Watson	1878–1958
Emil Kraepelin	1856–1926
Eugene Bleuler	1857–1939
Adolph Meyer	1866–1950

SOCIAL SCIENTISTS

Auguste Comte	1798–1851
Herbert Spencer	1820–1903
Emile Durkheim	1858–1917
Charles Cooley	1864–1929
George Mead	1863–1931
William I. Thomas	1863–1947
Edward Sapir	1884–1939
Ruth Benedict	1887–1948
Kurt Lewin	1890–1947

INTRAPERSONAL THEORISTS

Jean Martin Charcot	1825–1893
A. A. Liebeault	1823–1904
Hippolyte Bernheim	1837–1919
Pierre Janet	1859–1947
Josef Breuer	1842–1925
Sigmund Freud	1856–1939
Alfred Adler	1857–1939
Carl Jung	1875–1961
Otto Rank	1884–1940
Sandor Ferenzi	1873–1933
Wilhelm Reich	1897–1957

PHYSICISTS
(RELATIONSHIPS AND RELATIVITY)

Albert Michelson	1852–1931
Edward Morley	1833–1923
Albert Einstein	1879–1955
Sir Arthur Stanley Eddington	1882–1944
Neils Bohr	1885–1962
Erwin Schrodinger	1887–1961
Sir James Jeans	1877–1946
Max Born	1882–1970
Werner Heisenberg	1901–1976

INTERPERSONAL THEORISTS

Harry Stack Sullivan	1892–1949
Karen Horney	1885–1952
Clara Thompson	1893–1958
Frieda Fromm Reichman	1890–1957
Eric Fromm	
Trigant Burrow	1875–1951
Eric Berne	

NEURAL SUBSTRATE AND
INFORMATION THEORISTS

Sir Charles
Sherrington 1857–1952
M. W. Magoun
John C. Eccles
Roger Sperry
J. Z. Young
Charles Pribram
Joseph E. Bogen
Arthur J. Deikman
Robert E. Ornstein

FAMILY AND COMMUNICATION
THEORISTS

Gregory Bateson
Don Jackson
Jay Haley
Nathan Ackerman
Murray Bowen
Carl Whitaker
Virginia Satir
Theodore Lidz
Salvador Minuchin

LINGUISTS

Claude Levi-Strauss
Roger Brown
Benjamin Whorf
Noam Chomsky
L. S. Vygotsky

MATHEMATICIANS
(INFORMATION PROCESSING)

John Von Neumann 1903–1951
C. E. Shannon
Norbert Wiener

SYSTEMS THEORISTS

LEARNING THEORISTS

Jean Piaget
Konrad Lorenz
B. F. Skinner

Ludwig von Bertalanffy
James G. Miller
Anatol Rapoport
Roy Grinker
Karl Menninger
Harley Shands
George Engel
Jurgen Ruesch

CONTRIBUTORS IN
OTHER FIELDS

Igor Stravinsky	1882–1971
Pablo Picasso	1881–1973
Henry Ford	1863–1947
James Joyce	1882–1941

is arbitrary, and scholars would probably differ on the categories and the persons listed in them. Some of the theorists listed might be representative of more than one area of study. For example, most of the interpersonal theorists could be called family and communication theorists as well. The chart should, however, clarify what is happening with regard to system theories.

As we can see from the quote by Auguste Comte at the beginning of this chapter, the study of systems is not new but it has been difficult until recently to focus our attention on it.

In the words of Trigant Burrow,

> Scientists, however, have not yet accepted the full implication of an organismic position as it applies to man's interrelational behavior . . . [Although] the scientific world in general has turned more and more to the study of functioning wholes, the accustomed approach to man's behavior in relation to his fellows is still essentially atomistic. . . . In our feeling-life we are all isolationists. We are discrete and often conflicting entities, prejudiced in favor of the self and what we conceive to be its unilateral advantage [7, p. 63].

Even as man began to differentiate himself from the other animals, he pondered his role in nature. In this book, we have described the development of man's self system, the hunger of this self system for information, and the attempts of each self system to stay synchronous with its environment. Once man learned that he is a unique individual with the endowment of self-consciousness, he began to speculate as to his relationship with all other systems.

According to John C. Eccles,

> I would put the dawn of self-consciousness, the sure knowledge of World 2, as at least 100,000 years ago because the earliest known Neanderthal ceremonial graves were at that time. . . . We can surmise that at that time a primitive man would be looking at others dying and thinking, "He's like me. This can happen to me. I too can cease to live." And then began that transmutation from being just knowing creatures, to creatures that know that they know, which is the essence of self-consciousness [10, p. 220].

Early Philosophers and the Scientific Method

Although ancient literature addresses the subject of man's place in the universe, it is interwoven with supernatural and mythological expressions, which excludes it from the type of thinking that we presently term scientific. We will begin our present discussion with *Francis Bacon* (1561–1626) who has been given credit for initiating the scientific pattern of thinking.

Bacon argued that man was wasting his time trying to think up proofs of religious doctrines and that there should be a separation of philosophy and religion. He placed religious doctrines in a separate category, and began to turn his attention toward developing a manner of thinking that could give a more certain knowledge of the universe to mankind. The method that he developed is known as *induction*.

Bacon believed that by examining the similarities and differences among objects, man could then discover the forms, laws, or causes of such objects in the universe. In this way, man could explore the universe with some understanding. Bacon believed that the universe was composed of individual bodies and nothing else, and that these bodies acted according to definite and fixed laws. If one could understand the laws, then one would have the understanding to unravel all the mysteries and, eventually, would be able to control the universe. In effect, he deemphasized religion and moved toward laws. Bacon, however, did not denounce God. He recognized God as of primary importance but he emphasized observation of fixed laws as the way to complete understanding.

Thomas Hobbes (1588–1679) extended what Bacon had started, and severed completely with the past. Hobbes was a student of mathematics and, as he began to write about the world in terms comparable to mathematics, a new and modern era began in philosophy. Hobbes pointed out the similarities in men and felt that vanity allowed all men to think that they were different when, actually, the differences in intellectual and physical capacity were minimal. With wit and some degree of cynicism he argued that each man may claim that he knows there are others who are more intelligent, witty, and so on, than he is, but that, in his heart, he still believes himself to be superior in wisdom. Thus, he claimed, men are more equal than unequal since each person is content with his own lot in life, seeing himself secretly as being in possession of greater knowledge and understanding.

Hobbes wrote that every man wants as much as he can get, wants to keep what he gets secure, and wants other people to appreciate what he has accomplished. He believed that ethical qualities exist only in a social system and are not part of man's innate make-up. Therefore, Hobbes tended to leave ethics, religion, and other social mores out of this description and became one of the first major philosophers to address man objectively as an animal and as an animal in relationship to his culture.

Philosophers Concerned with Man and Nature

Following Hobbes, there were a number of philosophers who addressed the theme of man and his nature or man and Nature. *Rene Descartes* (1596–1650) separated man into mind and body (the psyche–soma dichotomy), and maintained that the mind was unable to influence the body, and the body was unable to influence the mind. They were totally separate. However, although they were separate, they both depended on God.

Since Descartes was also a mathematician, he was interested in building a theory that was logical and mechanistic. Descartes believed that all the laws of nature were laws of motion and that, if one thing speeded up, another thing must slow down, as there was only a certain amount of motion given by God to the universe. Because of the Cartesian dualism (separation of mind and body), some men began to speculate that there was no material world outside the mind of man, that man could know absolutely nothing about material things, since his mind was separate from them.

John Locke (1632–1740) was very much involved in the theories of Descartes. He accepted the mind–body dichotomy, but went on to reason that man's knowledge was all derived from sense impressions. Therefore, he stated, there must be a material world to give us these sense impressions. For example, we could not have the sensation of something being hard it there were not a hard substance in existence. Locke believed that the entire world was composed of substances, including body and soul, and that these substances could act upon each other and influence each other. Although he spoke of interaction, his philosophy was still considered akin to Descartes and the dualism of mind and body because he argued that although both soul and body were substances, they were different kinds of substances.

George Berkeley (1685–1753) completely eliminated, in his theories, the material universe. He argued that things were seen (for example, trees and flowers) because they existed in the mind. If a person walked away from a tree, the tree might still be there because it might be in the mind of another person who was looking at the tree. And if there was no one else there, the tree might still exist in the mind of God. Berkeley believed that the source of all our ideas was God and that man was able to see what God allowed him to see. All that existed was what man perceived. If he did not perceive a thing, it was not there.

David Hume (1711–1776) refused to believe in the existence of any substance at all. He stated that God did not exist and that all that man could be sure of was his own ideas. The ideas of man came one after the other but they did not stem from any source such as God. He did not know where ideas came from or where they went but he saw no reason for belief in either a world of substance or in God. The philosophy of Hume was totally mind centered.

Gottfried Wilhelm Leibnitz (1646–1716) built his philosophy around the idea of harmony in the universe. He believed that the universe was constructed of units of substance called *monads* and that they acted in harmony with each other. Man is also built of monads. Each monad acted according to the laws of God. God, having once constructed the monads, set everything in motion and then withdrew from the world. What happened to the world was then a matter of mechanics and the laws that governed the monads. This reinforced Bacon's thesis and gave great hope to scientific thinkers, because it implied a world of laws which could be discovered and that were fixed in nature.

At this point we can clearly visualize the coupling of two areas of thought (a) emphasis on man as a part of nature and (b) a growing reverence for nature as a perfect system. Man, even though he could study only his own thoughts, should try to harmonize those thoughts with nature. To find contradictions in the laws of nature would be to imply that an already perfect system was imperfect and would challenge the harmony or balance inherent in the basic paradigm.

If the universe was only in the mind of man, he could observe only his own ideas, for no material universe existed. If a material universe did exist, it was subject to fixed laws, already perfect, and unalterable by human thought or observation. Thus far, scientific and philosophical thought had served only to confuse all issues and led some individuals to distrust the motives and effects of further study. It seemed to some that it would be better to abdicate thought altogether.

For example, *Jean Jacques Rousseau* (1712–1778) advocated that man return to nature completely. He argued that man had been corrupted by science, culture, and learning. In order to reach his full potentialities, man must get out of civilization and all its corrupting influences. He believed that man was not mechanical but a creature of feeling and sentiment who could fully experience those feelings only under "natural" or more primitive conditions.

Philosophic thought seemed to have reached an impasse until *Immanuel Kant* (1725–1804) put forth yet another theory. Kant, a brilliant man who became known as a philosophical system-builder, admitted that knowledge was limited to ideas but, he stated, since man was able to reason, he could use his reasoning powers to act as if there were a universe surrounding him. He described the influence of perceptive ability on man's reason and thinking, and was one of the first to imply the limitations or relativity of man's ability to perceive his surroundings. In this rather clever compromise, he did not deny the importance of the human mind nor did he exclude the possibility of a universe interacting with that mind.

Johann Gottlieb Fichte (1772–1814) supported the work of Kant. He believed that man was part of what he called a *universal ego*. By this he seemed to imply that there was a universal mind of which the mind of man was only a part. The universe, which he described as the creative ego, had man as its highest expression. However, all objects (for example, rivers, mountains, and trees) were creations of the universal ego.

Arthur Schopenhauer (1788–1860) spoke of a universal will which, as he described it, was very similar to the phenomenon which Freud would subsequently describe as the id. This will (or id) was the permeating force that drove all life and perhaps nonlife to function, especially in reference to reproduction. This will had little concern for the individual person and was a driving blind force. Schopenhauer was criticized for being cynical. However, his writings increased the possibility of a scientific approach to the study of man.

Impact of the Work of Darwin   The world of philosophy and beginning science, particularly as related to the biologic sciences and the study of man, underwent a precipitous revolution and reorganization with the publication in 1858 of *The Origin of Species* by *Charles Darwin* (1809–1882). (We note the name of *Alfred Russel Wallace* [1823–1913] on the chart because

Wallace, an English naturalist, arrived at a very similar theoretical concept. Darwin's meticulous work in this area has resulted in his being given the most credit, while students remain unfamiliar with Wallace and his impressive contributions.)

Although the science of biology had been progressing, the study of man had been somewhat outside this perimeter until Darwin unequivocally stated that man was a mammal and on a continuum with the remainder of living organisms. The world of living organisms could no longer be viewed as a world of spontaneous creation, but as a world in process. Human behavior was no longer in the realm of philosophical study only but was open to examination by the biologic sciences. This view of man as being a product of evolution had tremendous impact upon the scientific world.

With the beginning of this new approach to the study of man came the development of two theoretical concepts in the study of human behavior, the intrapersonal and the interpersonal. Social scientists and anthropologists began to study human behavior in terms of its evolution as did the pragmatic, behaviorist, and descriptive theorists. Although these different views of man's behavior were not described in systems terms, they were all concerned with man as a set of systems within larger systems.

Intrapersonal Theorists   At about the same time that Darwin developed the theoretical concept of evolution, medicine—especially the neurologists—began to explore human behavior. They began to view the system of the individual and all its component parts with respect to effects on specific behaviors when alterations occurred within the central nervous system.

Jean Martin Charcot (1825–1893) was a French neurologist who is well known for his treatment of hysteria by hypnosis. Charcot documented the effect upon behavior of one person upon another through the power of suggestion. He concluded that persons who could be hypnotized must have some weakness that allowed them to succumb to the influence of another.

A. A. Liebault (1823–1904), a French country doctor, and *Hippolyte Bernheim* (1837–1919), his associate, worked with large numbers of peasants in Nancy, France, using the technique of hypnotic suggestion to alleviate their neurotic symptoms. Bernheim concluded that many so-called "normal" persons could be hypnotized, disputing Charcot's theory that only a weakness could allow hypnosis to be successful.

Pierre Janet (1859–1947), who had been influenced by Charcot's concepts, speculated about psychic energy and intellectual cohesiveness. He felt that emotional problems were due to a lack of cohesive power in the central nervous system, that is, the intellectual functioning.

Josef Breuer (1842–1925), a Viennese physician, was also involved in the scientific exploration of hysteria and collaborated with *Sigmund Freud* (1856–1939), an Austrian neurologist; in this area of research. Their findings were reported in 1895 in *Studies on Hysteria*.

Freud worked not only with Charcot and Breuer, but also with Liebault and Bernheim. He began development of the psychoanalytic technique as he became intensely involved with the cathartic therapy used to treat hysteria. The term *catharsis* in psychoanalysis is used to describe the technique of allowing patients to express any thoughts or feelings that come into their consciousness. This unscreened flow of information, or free association, gives the analyst clues concerning the data base of the patient's ego or self system. Freud and his disciples, including *Alfred Adler* (1857–1939), *Carl Jung* (1875–1961), *Otto Rank* (1884–1940), *Sandor Ferenzi* (1873–1933), and *Wilhelm Reich* (1897–1957) continually elaborated upon this investigatory technique for exploring the human mind. Freud is commonly referred to as the father of psychoanalysis.

Although the classic psychoanalytic school developed by these intrapersonal theorists did recognize the influence of culture on individual behavior, its main emphasis focused on instinctual drives and how the distortion of expression of these instinctual drives stemming from the id resulted in anxiety and emotional symptomotology. The id is a term used to designate that cauldron of unconscious instinctual energies, especially sexual energy (libido). Freud divided the instincts into two major categories: (*a*) those concerned with individual survival which he called the *ego instincts* and (*b*) those concerned with the species' survival which he termed *libidinal* (sexual) *instincts*.

It was Freud's conviction that ego instincts played little part in the development of neurosis (emotional problems), whereas blockage of species survival, that is, sexual or libidinal instincts, caused a great deal of anxiety and neurotic symptomotology. Those constrictions placed upon the expression of libidinal drive by society he termed *superego* (moral attitudes) and, since most of these constrictions were placed on the individual by the parents who were the socializing factors in a child's life, the superego to some degree represents an introjected or incorporated parental attitude.

In Freudian theory, the psychic apparatus is composed of three major components: (*a*) the id, which is the unconscious energizing instinctual system; (*b*) the superego, which is the cultural standard setting (ethical) system; and (*c*) the ego, which is that conscious part of the self system which mediates between the instinctual system (id) and the ethical system (superego).

Using systems terminology, we might say that Freud abstractly divided the human information-processing system into three major subsystems spanning biological and social data-processing paradigms.

Jung, in addition to his work with the psychoanalytic school, began to speculate about larger systems, and presented a concept that he termed the *collective unconscious*. He believed that individuals are influenced by psychic forces outside their awareness, which transcend cultures. These psychic influences are inherited and form the collective unconscious which unites cultural system.

Freud and his protégés developed an elaborate theoretical system explaining how behavioral patterns reflect the dynamic equilibrium between the conscious self (ego), the instinctual drives, and the restraint of cultural mores. Patterns that attempt to reconcile data that are dissynchronous with the self systems were termed *ego defense mechanisms*. Individuals were viewed as defending their self systems against change by behavioral techniques and attitudes called *character armor*. Reich is best known for his elaboration on dissecting out these patterns (character analysis).

Social Scientists   While the psychoanalysts were exploring intrapersonal psychic dynamics, there was a simultaneous movement in the field of sociology. This movement received little attention at the time, since it was not as explosively repulsive to the Victorian culture of that period.

Auguste Comte (1798–1851), a scientist and mathematician, theorized that all man could know was relationships. Everything must be interpreted in light of what he saw and experienced. He believed that, as man found regularity in his relationships, he could begin to predict what might happen and could work to change events accordingly.

Herbert Spencer (1820–1903), a utilitarian philosopher and civil engineer, saw man as a part of the evolutionary process. He also believed that man's experiences were the result of an activity or force which he termed the *unknowable,* which was the cause of all experiences and the fundamental principle of both man and the universe. Comte and Spencer are accredited as the first to address social phenomena scientifically.

Emile Durkheim (1858–1917), a contemporary of Freud's, proved to be a major force in the movement of the social scientists to explain the individual as a part of a social system. Durkheim was convinced that the individual must participate in a social system in his search for rationality and spirituality. He developed the theory of anomie or psychic pain. When a person feels that society is not exerting the controls necessary to give him the illusion of security, he begins to experience anomie.

Durkheim wrote of society as having an interdependency with the individual, as though society were an entity itself with a nature peculiar to itself. Society needed the individual to pursue its ends just as the individual needed society. He believed that society acted as an entity in (*a*) using moral authority and objects of respect such as a leader or a deity to maintain power over the individual, (*b*) enforcing conformity by the evolving of legal instruments, and (*c*) screening information among individuals within the society.

Durkheim also believed that moral authority was dependent upon public opinion. Once this moral authority was recognized and accepted, it had an enormous effect or influence on the thinking of any of the group's members. A classic example of this type of phenomena is seen in the experience of Galileo, whose theories were not accepted because they conflicted with the accepted moral authority of that time—the Inquisition.

It is interesting that Durkheim used a concept of psychic energy in describing the operational force of a cultural unit that was very similar to Freud's use of psychic energy in describing that of the individual. Durkheim felt that the psychic energy or force that acted upon man as a collective consciousness became introjected into the individual. He knew that he was being acted upon but he did not know by whom. Social forces became part of the individual's own self system. In addition, the collective consciousness had a self system or characteristics of its own as well as the characteristics of its unitized parts. Durkheim felt that it was a group who spoke through each individual.

Another sociologist who had major impact on the thinking of social scientists of this time was *Charles Cooley* (1864–1929). Cooley's work overlaps to some degree that of Durkheim's. Cooley also believed that the self system of the individual is fused with that of the group. He stated that each person is ambitious to achieve some desired position in the thoughts of others. Cooley implied that there was peer pressure for individuals to conform to the attitude of others in order to gain their respect and esteem. Cooley was the originator of the "looking glass theory," which stated simply that each person reflected each other person. He believed that human nature was group nature and that there was a social mind.

Cooley was an American sociologist and Durkheim, French. They developed their theories at about the same time. It would be difficult to say which was the more influential in the field of sociology and related fields.

Two other American sociologists, *George Mead* and *William I. Thomas,* both born in 1863 and contemporaries of Durkheim and Cooley, to some degree reiterated the immense influence that culture has on human behavior. Mead (1863–1931) is perhaps best known for his emphasis on *the internalized other*: The individual must develop the abstract capability of internalizing another person's attitude before he can fully develop his own self system. Everyone emits behaviors that evoke responses, and everyone responds to behaviors of others. Our responses are generally patterned after the responses of others. This is another way of saying that we are able to predict how people will respond to ourselves by putting ourselves in their position. Mead believed that language can have meaning only if we synchronize the effect of the language on others with the meaning it has for ourselves.

In speaking of internalized others, Mead emphasized that the individual does not internalize a concrete person but a system of relationships composed of role expectations both for the other person and for himself. Mead is perhaps the most emphatic in stating that we can understand ourselves only as a set of relationships to others. (In this, he antedates Sullivan, whose theories we will address later.) Mead stated without reservation that there can be no individual self without a society in which the person can assume the role of a generalized other in order to understand himself reflectively. This is very similar to Cooley's theory that we see ourselves through others, who more or less serve as mirrors or looking glasses for us.

Thomas (1863–1947) differed slightly in his emphasis. Although he, too, stated that individual behavior is greatly influenced by society, he believed that we can study behavior only by studying the forces that impel the individual to act. The action of social forces is evidenced in the form of human desires or wishes, which Thomas classified. He stated that each individual is driven by four different desires or wishes for four different things:

1. New experience.
2. Security.
3. Response.
4. Recognition.

In these categories there is some similarity to an earlier theory of Thomas Hobbes, in which he described man's need for competition, security and glory.

Thomas used his four categories to clarify different patterns of human behavior and to delineate different patterns of personality. He described some persons as being more aggressive in the need for excitement, and linked this need with creativity and other human endeavors such as sports. He described other persons as being more given to the desire for security. They may avoid the dangers of a new experience, retiring in a type of fight–flight pattern when placed in an insecure situation.

Thomas believed that the human animal continually desires attention for the development and maintenance of his self system. The individual acquires this attention and status from society alone. Society also forces the individual to conform in a covert way while conferring status upon him. Thomas implied an understanding of social reinforcement by stating that nature reinforces behavioral patterns through negative and positive appreciation. However, he tempered this behavioristic attitude by the theory that patterns of behavior are also influenced by the person's temperament. The interaction of social pressure and temperament form character.

Edward Sapir (1884–1939), an American anthropologist, sociologist and linguist, was one of the first to focus on language as a social instrument and how language itself distorted social operations and the individual's attitudes toward himself and his environment. *Ruth Benedict* (1887–1948), another anthropologist of the time, added diversity to cultural studies by focusing on differences among cultures, that is, the different patterns of culture and how these patterns influence different individual attitudes.

Two Major Theoretical Orientations   At the close of the nineteenth century and the beginning of the twentieth century, there were two major theoretical orientations toward the study of human behavior. The first was that of the psychoanalytic, or Freudian, school, whose major emphasis was on the id or instinctual drives of the individual as characterized by Freud's belief that the individual is "a short-lived appendage to a germ-plasm, an episode in a series of generations virtually insured of immortality [12, p. 263]." The main theme of this orientation was the attempt to view behavior as a biologic function. The emphasis in this conceptual paradigm was on individual constitution and psychic energy as the major forces influencing the individual behavioral readout. Freud did give credence to the self or ego, as he termed it, and described it as being analogous to the rider of a horse, whose function was to guide the power and energy of the basic libidinal drives. The ego was indeed developed from the id, as were some of the introjected cultural values that he termed superego. However, these were deemed of little importance unless they interfered with the flow of psychic energy, chief among which was sexual energy (libido).

In the second major school, catalyzed by Durkheim and elaborated by Cooley, Mead, and others, culture was conceptualized as the major guiding force in forming and maintaining a self or an ego. These scholars contested that there could be no awareness of an individual self without cultural input via the linguistic tools of society and that our "selves" must be mirrored by others in order for us to have any concept of being unique and different.

Pragmatic, Behaviorist, and Descriptive Theorists   In addition to those working in the two major schools of theoretical orientation just described, other scholars were making a contribution toward the understanding of human behavior that do not fit adequately into the two major classifications. *William James* (1842–1910),

American philosopher, physician, and psychologist who is considered by some to be America's most original philosopher, is perhaps best known for his emphasis on pragmatism. He was most concerned in his writing with trying to structure the energies and powers of men. He believed that men are as creative in their cognitive as in their active lives. In his words,

In our cognitive as well as in our active life we are creative. We add, both to the subject and to the predicate part of reality. The world stands really malleable, waiting to receive its final touches at our hand. Like the kingdom of heaven, it suffers violence willingly. Man engenders truths upon it [14, pp. 256–257].

John Dewey (1859–1952), American philosopher and educator, wrote extensively and incisively on pragmatism and on James' works. Both James and Dewey contended that pure theoretical formulation without functional correlation is of little value in understanding the human condition.

The emphasis placed by the pragmatists on the functional aspects of theory building was augmented by another group of scholars who addressed the manner or method by which man learns. *Ivan Pavlov* (1849–1936), a Russian neurophysiologist seven years older than Freud, almost serendipitously discovered a mode of addressing learning through the conditioned reflex. He helped to objectify the learning paradigms of animals, and was able to speculate about learning in humans. These speculations led him to address the various signal systems including the first and second signal system of man, the second being synonomous with abstract language or the symbolic operation. Today, Pavlov's name is associated with the term *conditioning,* and those who are familiar with his work refer to Pavlovian classical conditioning. It is of interest that Pavlov received a Nobel prize for his work on digestion prior to being recognized for the field of study most commonly referred to in standard texts of psychology as being associated with his name.

Conditioning is a type of learning in which physiologic phenomena are paired with stimuli. This opened the door for conceptualizing human behavior as a physiologic phenomenon that persists if reinforced by the internal or external milieu of the animal. The human aspect of man's behavior is a unique physiological activity that is socially reinforced. To reiterate this point, we stress that behavioral patterns are physiologic processes that are sustained as patterns via social reinforcement. This conceptualization falls neatly into the framework built by Pavlov as he studies classical conditioning.

John Watson (1878–1958), American psychologist, developed a conceptual frame that has been termed *behavioristic*. He implied that all behavior can be altered by changing the environment. Both Watson and Pavlov have contributed to understanding the stimulus–response paradigm and its relationship to learning.

At the same time that the social and behavioral theorists were at work, many clinicians were addressing the various patterns of behavior that they witnessed in their clinical activities. Two of the most notable of these were *Emil Kraepelin* (1856–1926) and *Eugen Bleuler* (1857–1939), both contemporaries of Freud who made lasting contributions in categorizing and classifying various patterns of behavior. These classifications continue to influence our present diagnostic nosology.

Kraepelin's methods were definitely objective, but they revolved only around the behaviors of the patient and did not consider the environment or the family. Kraepelin's observations did permit a clear differentiation between dementia praecox and manic-depressive psychosis. One unfortunate result of Kraepelin's observations was the belief that anyone classified as a victim of dementia praecox was considered incurable. It was Bleuler who first used the term *schizophrenia* when referring to dementia praecox. The word has a Greek derivation meaning "split mind" and refers to the dissociation between affects (emotions) and thoughts. Bleuler's writings leave a more hopeful view of the prognosis for schizophrenia than those of Kraepelin.

Another clinician who influenced American thinking to a great extent was *Adolph Meyer* (1866–1950). Meyer, a psychiatrist ten years younger than Freud, had a keen sense for social influences on behavior, but was well rooted in the biologic sciences as a neuropathologist. He developed a theoretical construct that he called *psychobiology*, which attempted to amalgamate biologic and social forces as vectors influencing human behavior.

Interpersonal Theorists   One of Meyer's pupils who accepted much of psychoanalytic theory but also had an expanded appreciation for social influences was *Harry Stack Sullivan* (1892–1949), whose name is almost synonymous with the interpersonal theory of psychiatry. Sullivan was much influenced by Cooley, Meade, Thomas, Sapir, and Benedict in the development of his theoretical formulations.

Sullivan and his colleagues, *Karen Horney* (1885–1952), *Clara Thompson* (1893–1958), *Frieda Fromm Reichman* (1890–1957), and *Eric Fromm* developed a rather loose and complex heuristic model for applying social concepts in formulating ideas about emotional problems and normal human development. This school of thought has been termed *neo-Freudian* or *interpersonal* as opposed to the classic intrapsychic model given by the Freudian school.

Freud had postulated that the distortion of sexual (libidinal) energies resulted in anxiety and neurosis. Sullivan postulated that distortion of ego activities resulted in emotional disturbances. He felt that a neurosis was the product of cultural environment, stemming from distorted interpersonal relationships rather than instincts. He implied that anxiety almost always stems from disapproval from others. The similarity between this approach and that of Cooley's looking glass theory is evident.

Sullivan used the term *self system* in a manner similar to Freud's use of the term ego. Sullivan believed that the individual self system forms from interpersonal experiences with others as the person tries to ameliorate the tensions arising from his drives or needs. The importance of others in the maintenance of a self system results in heavy emphasis on family dynamics.

An example of the difference between Sullivan and Freud might be seen in the interpretation of the classic Oedipal conflict. From a Freudian approach the emphasis is on the child's ability to negotiate his instinctual drives toward parents of the same and opposite sex. In the Sullivanian, or interpersonal, theory, the emphasis would be on the parental attitudes toward the child and the child's reciprocal response. In this paradigm, the father would respond differently to a male child than to a female child so that the Oedipal conflict is an interaction or an interpersonal phenomenon rather than a biologic or instinctually motivated behavioral process. Sullivan explained this by saying that parents identify with their child of the same sex and have different expectations for it than for the child of the opposite sex.

Trigant Burrow (1875–1951), a psychoanalyst who was one of those responsible for the introduction of psychoanalysis to the United States, is mentioned in this section because of his departure from the traditional analytic approach, which emphasized individualism. Burrow became increasingly convinced that human behavior must be studied in the context of the group and the interpersonal behaviors among individuals. Consequently, he developed a conceptual frame known as *phyloanalysis,* which stressed an organismic frame of reference and the study of behavior through the observation of group dynamics.

Eric Berne has had tremendous impact upon the field of human behavior, with his emphasis on *transactional analysis* as a group treatment technique. He developed a transactional theory of personality and is especially noted for his study of group dynamics and the classifying of various games people play in interpersonal relationships.

Family and Communication Theorists
With the emphasis on interpersonal relationships, many scholars began to concentrate on the study of families and communications patterns within families. *Gregory Bateson* was emphatic in stressing the point that any scientific study must confront the problem of complex interacting systems and subsystems. In his words, "It followed that all directional change, even in biological evolution and phylogeny, might—or must—be due to progressive interaction between organisms [2, p. 155]." He extended his study of interaction to the evolution of the "contexts" of behavior, and was especially interested in the communication systems in the families of alcoholics and schizophrenics.

Don Jackson is considered one of the foremost innovators in developing family interactional psychotherapy. He was instrumental in promoting the idea that all family members should be present for any therapy session. He modified this stance later to the idea that different combinations of family members could be treated. All treatment, however, must be considered effectual only if done in the context of the family and related subsystems such as fellow students or colleagues. In other words, the patient is seen as a member, not only of family, but of various other groups.

Jay Haley and others attempted to quantify information exchanged within families and to establish rules by which roles and counterroles interacted, and the mode by which relationships were defined. Haley described relationships as being either symmetrical or complementary, depending upon whether the participants were of equal control or in a passive–dominant relationship.

Nathan Ackerman was another of the pioneers in the attempt to promote family therapy rather than individual therapy. His clinical work and his writing centered on family diagnosis and treatment. In 1958, he wrote,

The investigation of the psychodynamics of the family as a unit and the processes of individual integration into the family group, previously neglected, opens up a new avenue of research. The relations of individual personality and the group-dynamic processes of family living constitute an essential link in the chain of causation of states of mental illness and health [1, pp. 24–25].

Murray Bowen developed his own family systems theory and pioneered efforts to look at multiparty information exchange. He described triangulation as a form of communication and interpersonal control.

Carl Whitaker was instrumental in the development of a family network therapy and the study of the family as a four-dimensional relationship.

Virginia Satir is the scholar most closely associated with *conjoint family therapy*. Most of her contributions revolve around the use of insight in changing communication patterns.

Theodore Lidz described "family schism" and "family skew" to delineate disjointed information flow in disturbed families.

Salvador Minuchin and his colleagues studied patterns of family dysfunction and concentrated upon methods to disrupt those dysfunctional patterns. For example, they described treatment methods for chronic asthma that took into account family roles and family structures. Minuchin is the foremost proponent of *structural family therapy*, and has written extensively on that subject.

Physicists (Relationships and Relativity)
From Francis Bacon's search in the 1500s for the laws that govern the universe to the family and communication theorists and their search for the keys to interpersonal communication, the evolution toward a systems approach to the study of human behavior is evident. At the turn of this century, studies in sociology, psychology, and biology were reorganizing a conceptual frame for understanding man. There was a growing awareness that man could not be separated from his environment. The study of man must, therefore, include his cybernetic interaction with all the phenomena surrounding him. This view was enormously reinforced by revolutionary concepts that burst on the scene in nuclear physics and

astrophysics. These concepts deal specifically with relativity and the relationship of events.

In 1887 *Albert Michelson* (1852–1931) and *Edward Morley* (1833–1923) carried out an experiment that rocked the physicists and questioned Newton's laws. Their experiment concerned the direction and speed of light. It is unclear whether or not *Albert Einstein* (1879–1959) was familiar with that experiment, but he continued asking questions about light and the speed of light that led to his relativity theories.

In any discussion of the impact of physics upon our world view, the name of Einstein is preeminent. Every philosophical approach to science has undergone change as a result of his formulations. His conceptualization of the relativity and interdependency of the phenomena we term time, space, mass and energy catalyzed a complete reorganization of our world view with even more dramatic implications than Darwin's theories. The concept of relativity shifted scientific attention to events and functions instead of objects and forms.

Sir Arthur Stanley Eddington (1882–1944), a British astronomer, studied the motions of the stars, relativity, and stellar evolution. He was convinced that it was now possible for the scientific community to become reconciled with the religious community, and tried to apply the concepts being formed in physics to human experience.

Eddington's writing inspired new conceptual frames. For example, he described the atoms of a table in relationship to the atoms of his body in a way that indicates continual overlapping systems extending from galaxies to the force fields of atoms that make up man and his universe. He wrote,

> To reach the reality of the table we need to be endowed with sense-organs to weave images and illusions about it. And so it seems to me that the first step in a broader revelation to man must be the awakening of image-building in connection with the higher faculties of his nature, so that these are no longer blind alleys but open out into a spiritual world—a world partly of illusion, no doubt, but in which he lives no less than in the world, also of illusion, revealed by the atom [11, pp. 454–455].

Eddington openly expresses a sense of reverence for the scintillating relationships among the systems that make up man and his environment.

Neils Bohr (1885–1962), 1922 Nobel prize winner in physics, introduced to physics a new model of the atom.

Bohr presented the atom as a dynamic–harmonic system. We include him here, not only because he was one of the greatest of the turn-of-the-century physicists, but because he accomplished his revolutionary concept by synthesizing Rutherford's concept of the atom with Max Planck's quantum theory. This conceptual amalgamation, which has been enormously productive in subsequent studies in physics, stemmed from Bohr's appreciation of relationships. He emphasized that language can never be totally accurate and that in dealing with fluid relationships we are limited to analogies.

Erwin Schrodinger (1887–1961), 1933 Nobel prize winner in physics, was interested not only in the quantum theory and wave mechanics but in the relationship between culture and science. He said that to look at "strictly causal connections" was to be too limited and that this was the error often made by the scientist. His caution against placing events in a cause-and-effect sequence is extremely pertinent to those scholars who study sequential human behavior.

Sir James Jeans (1877–1946), British physicist, related modern concepts in physics to the questions of free will and determinism. He emphasized that the new physics had emphatically decided the question of whether we can fully comprehend the realities of nature. We cannot, he concluded, and all we can really study is our own observations. He believed that our "prison walls" of time and space keep us from learning that which is beyond time and space. His writings are rather reminiscent of the early philosophers even though his field of study was modern stellar dynamics and radiation.

Max Born (1882–1970) wrote that theoretical physics and philosophy are synonymous. He concentrated not on a world of objects, but on a world of interactions. The world interacts with the viewer and cannot be separated from the viewer. Each person must interpret his own perceptions.

One of Born's pupils, *Werner Heisenberg* (1901–1976), developed what is accepted as being one of the most profound scientific concepts of the twentieth century, the *principle of uncertainty*. No "object" is ever exact. It is only similar to what it looked like when viewed before. Everything is changing, and the very act of looking at an object or event changes it. This conceptual viewpoint had enormous impact upon the study of human behavior. The process of studying behavior alters that behavior. Every interaction produces change. The physicists have continued to make startling discoveries that emphasize the importance of studying relationships and functions rather than objects. So far, they have not been able to delineate a closed system. Those scientists in the field of human behavior who have been moving steadily toward seeing man as a set of systems within larger systems can find in modern physics an ally of some consequence.

Neural Substrate and Information Theorists

Any study of man's behavior must address the human brain. Until the middle of the nineteenth century, the brain was seen as an organ, perhaps the major organ, associated with human perception, motor activity, thought, and communication. Most studies were directed toward the complex anatomical structures composing the brain. The emphasis on form began to give way to consideration of function as scientists realized this master organ was a system composed of a multitude of subsystems with interacting and interdependent functions.

Sir Charles Sherrington (1857–1952), one of the great scientists of the nineteenth and twentieth centuries, emphasized the distortion inherent in the mind–body dichotomy and the necessity of studying the brain as a system with all its subsystems. He wrote poetically of the brain and of the search of man for the location of the human mind. He described the activity within the brain while a person is sleeping and as a person begins to wake. He writes,

> The great topmost sheet of the mass, that where hardly a light had twinkled or moved, becomes now a sparkling field of rhythmic flashing points with trains of travelling sparks hurrying hither and thither. The brain is waking and with it the mind is returning. It is as as if the Milky Way entered upon some cosmic dance. Swiftly the head-mass becomes an enchanted loom where millions of flashing shuttles weave a dissolving pattern though never an abiding one; a shifting harmony of subpatterns [17, pp. 177–178].

Sherrington was not only a scientist but a writer whose book *Man on His Nature* is an inspiring account of his search for answers to the mystery of the human brain. He could perhaps be called one of the earliest of the systems theorists because of his emphasis upon patterns and subpatterns, upon function as well as form. He agreed with the physicists that we will never know the answers but can only direct our attention to the search for more information.

H. W. Magoun has made a major contribution to the field of brain research in being able to delineate the anatomical and physiological systems (reticular activating system) associated with states of arousal, that is, sleeping, waking, and attentiveness. He has given us new information concerning the relationship of behavior and brain function that adds to the data base of several disciplines including psychology, psychiatry, philosophy, neurology, and education.

John C. Eccles, who has done pioneering work concerning information processing at the neuronal level, gives a short and intriguing account of brain research in *The Understanding of the Brain,* which is of interest to those in many disciplines. He discusses the relationship of brain, speech, and consciousness and the impact of brain research upon philosophy and psychology as well as physiology.

Eccles has made significant contributions by attempting to make the study of the brain as simple as possible for students and by emphasizing that the human self is a dynamic interaction of multiple systems.

Numbers of scholars are now studying those systems of the brain concerned with the physiologic paradigm by which perceptive inputs are coded and associated within the central nervous system and the difference between functions in the right and left hemispheres of the brain. Some of their work indicates that the right and left hemisphere functions are roughly analogous to the analog and digital processes, which helps us appreciate the abstracting or symbolic operation of human data processing.

Included among the major researchers in this area are *Roger Sperry, J. Z. Young,* and *Charles Pribram.* Sperry did extensive research with human subjects whose right and left hemispheres were separated. He hypothesized about the complementary functions of these hemispheres, with the left (dominant) hemisphere being more involved in linguistic (digital) operations and the right (nondominant) hemisphere being involved in the organization of data in a hologram of maplike gestalt (analog). Young referred to these functions with the terms *abstract* and *maplike.* Pribram used the same terminology we have adopted, analog and digital.

Joseph E. Bogen, a neurologist, is of primary importance because of his research in right–left hemisphere functions, which indicates that the two hemispheres process information differently. He theorized that the right hemisphere works simultaneously in processing data while the left hemisphere works through sequential thought. His work further indicates the productivity of using a bimodal model in studying human thought.

Arthur J. Deikman, a psychiatrist, is conducting research into altered states of consciousness, especially those which occur during meditation. He addresses the two modes of consciousness as the active and receptive, and contends that the receptive mode is essential to the development of man's highest potentialities and should not be devalued as the "lesser" of the two major modes.

Robert E. Ornstein, a research psychologist at the Langley Porter Neuropsychiatric Institute, has written and edited several books concerning the rational functions of the linear (left) hemisphere of the brain and the intuitive functions of the nonlinear (right) hemisphere. He has also investigated and analyzed Eastern and Western thought with respect to the right–left brain.

Learning Theorists   Another group of scholars that has contributed to our understanding of the way behavioral patterns develop are the learning theorists. This group is perhaps best exemplified by *Jean Piaget,* a Swiss psychologist, who, through personal observation, described children's ability to organize data at various stages of development. Piaget's studies of children illustrate that such concepts as space, quantity, time, and logic are developed by certain processes unique to each individual and are not totally preset attributes of the child's central nervous system.

Konrad Lorenz and other ethologists indicate that there is a critical time in the learning process for a young animal to incorporate certain patterns of behavior into its personal repertoire of activities. Exactly how this pertains to the human individual is as yet unexplored, although this work illustrates the need for role models in order for the individual to develop patterns similar to others of its species. This type of learning has been termed *imprinting* and has been validated with the work with finches and other species whose vocalizations are regulated by their dominant hemispheres.

B. F. Skinner, a behavioral psychologist, and his followers are noted for their studies of the effects of environmental manipulation as they applied instrumental conditioning to human learning. These experimenters decide what responses they wish to elicit from the individual and then attempt to "shape" the subject's actions by environmental manipulation so that he begins to move closer to the desired terminal behavior.

Linguists Linguists are making enormous contributions to the study of interpersonal relationships and the role of speech in the differentiation of man from all other animals. Evidence presented by various linguists seems to indicate that it is the structure of the brain, rather than its size, that makes the human brain human.

Claude Levi-Strauss, an anthropologist, placed heavy emphasis upon the work of the linguists and its application to anthropology. He stressed the importance of trying to find universal laws in the study of human nature just as the linguists try to find fundamental patterns in languages. He indicates the presence of information codes within the human brain and believes that it is the biological structure of the mind that has as its function the initiation of behavior. He emphasizes the importance of a systems approach in his belief that,

one must study the unconscious infrastructure of cultural phenomena rather than their surface manifestations; one must treat not the terms of units of the realm, but rather the relationships between those units, as independent entities; one must regard the entire domain as a system, and search for general laws, using the methods both of induction and of deduction [13, p. 119].

Roger Brown, a professor of social psychology, has written extensively in the field of psycholinguistics and has accomplished much toward bringing the behavioral sciences closer together in those areas concerned with language. He places special importance upon the idea that language is a system and states that, "Properly classified, linguistics seems to be a subdivision of cultural anthropology, for the linguist describes one kind of cultural system [6, p. xi]."

Benjamin Whorf has made comparative studies of various languages such as the Standard Average European which he refers to as the SAE and the Hopi. He also stresses that language is a system and concludes that such concepts as time, space, and matter are determined by the "nature of the language or languages through the use of which they have been developed [20, p. 148]."

Noam Chomsky has introduced a controversial theory which indicates that data processing as related to linguistic skills may be innate, at least in terms of its syntactic organization.

L. S. Vygotsky studied the relationship between thought and word and describes this relationship as a living process.

Thought and language, which reflect reality in a way different from that of perception, are the key to the nature of human consciousness. Words play a central part not only in the development of thought but in the historical growth of consciousness as a whole. A word is a microcosm of human consciousness [19, pp. 212–213].

Mathematicians   Refinements of the approaches to systems and information processing have been derived from technological advances in the computer sciences, and are characterized by the work of mathematicians including *C. E. Shannon, John von Neumann,* and *Norbert Wiener.* Wiener's introduction of the theories concerning cybernetics, that is, information used as a feedback mechanism for influencing subsequent information, has been of enormous value in understanding human learning.

Shannon became involved in the study of the central nervous system and its digital and analogic functions, including the construction of language. He proposed and proved several mathematical theorems concerning communication. Shannon is credited with the development of concepts, measures, and theorems known as *information theory,* which he initially applied to communication engineering. Information theory is now used in several other fields, for example, music.

Von Neumann, considered by many to be a genius and a mathematical prodigy as a child, developed a theory of games in which he took into consideration the "human" element, specifying that human behavior in "real life" is not like playing a game of chess, where there is eventually a solution but is a matter of deception and bluffing and trying to outguess the other person. His game theories emphasize the complexity of human information-processing systems. He formulated several mathematical theories of information processing. Von Neumann wrote a series of lectures which were published in 1956 in *The Computer and the Brain.* According to an analysis of these lectures by Bronowski, Von Neumann "looks at the brain as having a language in which the activities of the different parts of the brain have somehow to be interlocked and made to match so that we devise a plan, a procedure, as a grand overall way of life—what in the humanities we would call a system of values [5, p. 433]."

Wiener, Shannon, and Von Neumann were all interested and involved in cybernetics, and discussed together the digital and analogic components of information processing in the human brain and in the computer. One of their discussions can be read in *Cybernetics* published in 1951 and edited by Heinz von Foerster.

Contributors in Other Fields

The impetus toward a systems approach has not been confined to those fields we generally categorize as scientific. Enormous evolutionary changes have also been taking place in other fields, such as music, art, business, and literature.

Igor Stravinsky (1882–1971), a Russian composer, shocked the world with his new sounds for the symphony and with a different kind of mathematical composition, which allowed unusual combinations of tones and instruments. At first, his music was rejected because of the unfamiliarity of its harmonic and tonal qualities but it has gradually won acclaim and is now performed by major symphony orchestras throughout the world. Stravinsky approached the orchestra as a mathematical system with numerous digital combinations, just as previous composers had done, but he used tonal values and progressions that had not been used before.

Modern physics had, as one of its companions, modern art (5). The twentieth century artist began to look at geometrical designs and structure. *Pablo Picasso* (1881–1973) one of the inventors of cubism, was inspired by crystals and their formations, and began to paint mathematical shapes and to look for the structure underlying the surface of his subjects. The cubists no longer painted only from the idea of color and surface appearance, but looked for previously unappreciated rhythmic harmonies. Their works were a creation of the inner mind, a recreation of form through logical analysis. The modern or abstract artists began to utilize a different kind of information processing. Just as the physicist utilized the quantum, Picasso and others employed the cube as a unit of construction.

The writings of Freud had tremendous impact upon some of the twentieth century literary figures, who began to describe their characters as persons influenced by the "unconscious." *James Joyce* (1882–1941) is thought to be one of the writers who broke most completely with the literary traditions of the past. His *Ulysses* is a digitalization of an unconscious analogic gestalt in which he wrote through fragmentation. The relationship among these fragments and units must be understood in order to appreciate his novel as a system. Joyce also made some effort to translate music into prose.

Industry was also undergoing changes of enormous magnitude. *Henry Ford* (1863–1947) is credited for the development of the modern assembly line as a system. His emphasis upon the concept of the standardization of the interchangeability of these standardized units revolutionized industry. The systems that Ford created are still being used in the factories of today, and have allowed significant changes in our style of living and in our economy.

Systems Theorists   The vast amount of data now arriving from multiple sources and influencing theories of human behavior caused many of the previous theories to seem unilateral or limited in incorporating various types of information. Although psychologists had attempted to amalgamate existing theories of behavior through the use of organismic or gestalt psychology, the first serious attempt to use the concepts of wholeness and unity in biology was made in 1933 with the publication of *Modern Theories of Development: An Introduction to Theoretical Biology* by *Ludwig von Bertalanffy*. This book presented the conceptualization which von Bertalanffy hoped would provide a unifying paradigm not only for biology but for all related physiologic and health systems (3).

General systems theory has received overwhelming acceptance in the biologic sciences and is beginning to receive acceptance in the study of human behavior. Many other scholars are now making contributions in developing and modulating this theoretical frame to fit the study of human behavior. One of the most prominent theoreticians is *James G. Miller*, whose study of living systems is making an impact upon the behavioral sciences. His book *Living Systems* is a tremendous achievement in that it applies the same model to the study of the cell as well as to the study of supranational systems.

Anatol Rapoport is one of the foremost proponents of general systems theory as a tool for the reorganization of our thinking. He wrote

It [general systems theory] has revived the role of speculative analogy, more sophisticated, one would hope, than the naive analogies pursued by prescientific philosophers, deriving intellectual nourishment from advanced ideas of science. It has revived organismic thinking as a complement to analytic thinking, has suggested concepts appropriate to a holistic approach to both a conception of reality and to a theory of cognition [15, p. 237].

Roy Grinker has studied the relationship of symbolism, psychoanalytic theory, and general systems theory. *Karl Menninger* advocates the use of a holistic approach to the study of human behavior through the utilization of organization or systems theory. *Harley Shands* views a unified approach of all sciences to the study of human behavior as ideal. He wrote, "The three fields of neurophysiology, psychiatry, and sociology are bound together by the common factor that they are all concerned with the movement of coded information [16, p. 3]."

George Engel proposes that the use of a general systems approach to the study of human behavior will improve communication among the many disciplines involved. He advocates a biopsychosocial model as a new framework for teaching, research, and the delivery of health care.

Jurgen Reusch has been instrumental in developing a list of the minimal requirements for a general systems theory of human behavior.

Systems theory is the culmination and extension of multiple theories in fields of study ranging from atomic and astrophysics to interpersonal and international diplomacy. It allows an appreciation of the continuum of information processing whether the information be coded in force fields, ionic, molecular codes, electrical and hormonal intercellular codes, or in the complex linguistic codes of social operations. With systems theory, it is possible to address data organized within an atom, a molecule, a single cell, within an individual, in a family unit, an entire cultural or international system or stellar and planetary relationships in the universe. This theoretical approach will undoubtedly receive increasing attention in the ensuing decades.

> One is led to a new notion of unbroken wholeness which denies the classical idea of analyzability of the world into separately and independently existing parts. . . . We have reversed the usual classical notion that the independent "elementary parts" of the world are the fundamental reality, and that the various systems are merely particular contingent forms and arrangements of these parts. Rather, we say that inseparable quantum interconnectedness of the whole universe is the fundamental reality, and that relatively independently behaving parts are merely particular and contingent forms within this whole.
>
> David Bohm, 1975 (4)

> Quantum theory forces us to see the universe not as a collection of physical objects, but rather as a complicated web of relations between the various parts of a unified whole.
>
> Fritjof Capra, 1975 (8)

References   1. Ackerman, N. *The psychodynamics of family life: Diagnosis and treatment of family relationships*. New York: Basic Books, 1958.

2. Bateson, G. *Steps to an ecology of mind*. New York: Ballantine Books, 1972.

3. Bertalanffy; L. von, General systems theory and psychiatry—An overview. In W. Gray, F. Duhl, and N. Rizzo (Eds.), *General systems and psychiatry*. Boston: Little, Brown, 1969. Pp. 33–46.

4. Bohm, D. and Hiley, B. On the intuitive understanding of nonlocality as implied by quantum theory. *Foundations of Physics*, 1975, Vol. 5, pp. 96, 102.

5. Bronowski, J., *The ascent of man*. Boston: Little, Brown, 1973.

6. Brown, R. *Words and things: An introduction to language*. New York: Free Press, 1958.

7. Burrow, T. *Science and man's behavior*. New York: Philosophical Library, 1953.

8. Capra, F. *The tao of physics*. Boulder, Colorado: Shambhala, distributed in the U.S. by Random House, 1975, p. 138.

9. Comte, A. *The positive philosophy*, translated by H. Martineau. London: Bell, 1896, pp. 212–298.

10. Eccles, J. *The understanding of the brain*. New York: McGraw-Hill, 1973.

11. Eddington, Sir A. S. Reality, causation, science, and mysticism. In S. Commins and R. Linscott (Eds.), *Man and the universe: The philosophers of science*. New York, Washington Square Press, 1969.

12. Freud, S. *Introductory Lectures on Psychoanalysis,* Trans. Joan Riviere. London, Allen and Unwin, 1922.

13. Gardner, H. *The quest for mind.* New York: Vintage Books, 1974.

14. James, W. *Pragmatism: A new name for some old ways of thinking.* New York: Longman's Green, 1947.

15. Rapoport, A. General systems theory: A bridge between two cultures. *Behavioral Science,* 1976, *21,* 228–239.

16. Shands, H. C., *Thinking and psychotherapy: An inquiry into the processes of communication.* Cambridge, Massachusetts: Harvard University Press, 1960.

17. Sherrington, Sir C. *Man on his nature.* New York: Cambridge University Press, 1963.

18. Spencer, H. *The principles of sociology.* New York: Appleton, 1898, pp. 447–597.

19. Vygotsky, L. Thought and word. In P. Adams (Ed.), *Language in thinking.* Hammondsport, England: Penguin Books, 1972. Pp. 180–213.

20. Whorf, B. The relation of habitual thought and behavior to language. In P. Adams (Ed.), *Language in thinking.* Hammondsport, England: Penguin Books, 1972. Pp. 123–149.

Suggested Readings

Adams, P. (Ed.), *Language in thinking.* Hammondsport, England: Penguin Books, 1972.

Berne, E., *Games people play.* New York: Grove Press, 1964.

Berne, E., *Principles of group treatment.* New York: Oxford University Press, 1966.

Bronowski, J. *A sense of the future.* Cambridge, Massachusetts: MIT Press, 1977.

Brown, R. *Psycholinguistics: Selected papers.* New York: Free Press, 1970.

Butzer, K. Environment, culture, and human evolution. *American Scientist,* 1977, *65,* 572–584.

Calvin, M. Chemical evolution. *American Scientist,* 1975, *63,* 169–177.

Chomsky, N. *Language and mind.* New York: Harcourt Brace Jovanovich, 1968.

Clark, R., *Einstein: The life and times.* New York: Avon, 1972.

Commins, S., and Linscott, R. (Eds.), *Man and the universe: The philosophers of science.* New York: Washington Square Press, 1969.

Darwin, C. *Evolution and natural selection: An anthology of the writings of Charles Darwin* (B. Loewenberg, Ed.). Boston: Beacon Press, 1959.

Darwin, C., *The origin of species.* New York: Mentor, New American Library, 1958.

Deikman, A. *Personal freedom: On finding your way to the real world,* New York: Viking Press (Grossman), 1976.

Dimond, S., and Beaumont, J. (Eds.) *Hemisphere function in the human brain,* New York: Wiley (Halsted), 1974.

Engel, G. The need for a new medical model: A challenge for biomedicine. *Science,* 1977, *196*(4286), 129–136.

Ferguson, E. The mind's eye: Nonverbal thought in technology. *Science,* 1977, *197*(4306), 827–836.

Foerster, Heinz von, *Cybernetics.* New York: Josiah Macy, Jr. Foundation, 1951.

Freedman, A., Kaplan, H., and Sadock, B. (Eds.), *Modern synopsis of comprehensive textbook of psychiatry/II.* Baltimore: Williams and Wilkins, 1976.

Frost, S. E., Jr. *Ideas of the great philosophers: A survey of their basic teachings.* New York: Barnes and Noble, 1942.

Gray, W., Duhl, F., and Rizzo, N. (Eds.), *General systems theory and psychiatry.* Boston: Little, Brown, 1969.

Greenberg, G. The family interactional perspective: A study and examination of the work of Don D. Jackson. *Family Process,* 1977, *16*(4), 385–412.

Guerin, P. *Family therapy: Theory and practice.* New York: Gardner Press, 1976.

Haley, J. *Strategies of psychotherapy.* New York: Grune and Stratton, 1963.

Hamilton, V., and Vernon, M. (Eds.), *The development of cognitive processes.* New York: Academic Press, 1976.

Jackson, D. *Communication, family and marriage,* Palo Alto, California: Science and Behavior Books, 1970.

Jackson, D. *Therapy, communication, and change.* Palo Alto, California: Science and Behavior Books, 1970.

Kolb, L. *Modern clinical psychiatry.* Philadelphia: W. B. Saunders, 1977.

Lieder, P., Lovett, R., and Root, R. (Eds.). *British poetry and prose.* New York: Houghton Mifflin, 1950.

Magoun, H. *The waking brain.* Springfield, Illinois: Charles C Thomas, 1958.

McDermott, J. (Ed.), *The writings of William James.* New York: Random House, 1967.

Menninger, K., with Martin, M. and Pruyser, P., *The vital balance.* New York: Viking Press, 1963.

Miller, J., Living systems: Basic concepts. *Behavioral Science,* 1965, *10*(3), 193–237.

Miller, J., *Living systems.* New York: McGraw-Hill, 1978.

Oldfield, R., and Marshall, J. (Eds.), *Language.* Hammondsport, England: Penguin Books, 1968.

Ornstein, R. (Ed.), *The nature of human consciousness: A book of readings*. New York: Viking Press, 1974.

Ornstein, R. *The psychology of consciousness*. New York: Viking, 1972.

Parsons, T., Shils, E., Naegele, K., and Pitts, J. (Eds.). *Theories of society: Foundations of modern sociological theory*, Vols. I and I. New York: Free Press, 1961.

Piaget, J. *Insights and illusions of philosophy*. New York: World, 1971.

Piaget, J. *The origins of intelligence in children*. New York: Norton, 1963.

Popper, K., and Eccles, J. *The self and its brain*. New York: Springer International, 1977.

Richardson, E. *A short history of painting in America*. New York: Crowell, 1963.

Shands, H. *Semiotic approaches to psychiatry*. The Hague: Mouton, 1970.

Weisskopf, V. The frontiers and limits of science. *American Scientist*, 1975, *65*, 405–411.

Werley, H., Zuzich, A., Zajkowski, M., and Zagornik, A. (Eds.). *Health research: The systems approach*. New York: Springer, 1976.

Index